MEDICAL APHORISMS

TREATISES 1–5

THE MEDICAL WORKS
OF MOSES MAIMONIDES

Medical Aphorisms: Treatises 1–5

On Asthma

◆ ◆ ◆

Forthcoming Titles

Abridgments of the Works of Galen

Commentary on Hippocrates' Aphorisms

Medical Aphorisms: Treatises 6–10

Medical Aphorisms: Treatises 11–15

Medical Aphorisms: Treatises 16–20

Medical Aphorisms: Treatises 21–25

Medical Aphorisms: Indexes and Glossaries

On Asthma, Volume 2

On Coitus

On Hemorrhoids

On Poisons and the Protection against Lethal Drugs

The Regimen of Health

Maimonides

Medical Aphorisms
Treatises 1–5

كتاب الفصول في الطبّ

A parallel Arabic-English edition
edited, translated, and annotated by

Gerrit Bos

◆ ◆ ◆

PART OF THE MEDICAL WORKS
OF MOSES MAIMONIDES

Brigham Young University Press ◆ Provo, Utah ◆ 2004

LIBRARY OF CONGRESS CATALOGUING-IN-PUBLICATION DATA

Maimonides, Moses, 1135–1204.
[Kitāb al-fuṣūl fī al-ṭibb. Treatises 1–5. English & Arabic]
Maimonides medical aphorisms. Treatises 1-5 = Kitāb al-fuṣūl fī al-ṭibb : a parallel Arabic-English edition / edited, translated, and annotated by Gerrit Bos.
p. cm.—(The medical works of Moses Maimonides)
Includes bibliographical references and index.
ISBN 0–934893–75–6 (alk. paper)
1. Medicine—Aphorisms. [DNLM: 1. Aphorisms and Proverbs. 2. Philosophy, Medical. WZ 290 M223k 2004] I. Title: Kitāb al-fuṣūl fī al-ṭibb. II. Title: Medical aphorisms. III. Bos, Gerrit, 1948– IV. Title. V. Series.
R128.3. M62513 2004
610—dc22 2004001387

PRINTED IN THE UNITED STATES OF AMERICA.

1 2 3 4 5 6 7 8 9 10 09 08 07 06 05 04

First Edition

To Cees Peters

In Fond Memory

Contents

❖ ❖ ❖

Kitāb al-fuṣūl fī al-ṭibb (Medical Aphorisms)

◆ ◆ ◆

Sigla and Abbreviations

Arabic Manuscripts

G Gotha, orient. 1937, fols. 6–273.

G¹ Note in the margin of G.

L Leiden 1344, Or. 128,1 fols. 1–140.

L¹ Note in the margin of L.

P Paris, Bibliothèque nationale, héb. 1210, fols. 1–130.

E Escorial, Real Bibliotheca de El Escorial 868, fols. 117–26.

S Escorial, Real Bibliotheca de El Escorial 869, fols. 176–1.

S¹ Note above the line in S.

B Oxford, Bodleian, Uri 412, Poc. 319, cat. Neubauer 2113, fols. 1–123.

O Oxford, Bodleian, Hunt. Donat 33, Uri 423, cat. Neubauer 2114, 78 fols.

Hebrew Translations

ב *Medical Aphorisms,* Hebrew translation by Zeraḥyah ben Isaac Ben She'altiel Ḥen, MS Berlin, Or. Qu 512, (15th century), 280 pp.

מ *Medical Aphorisms,* Hebrew translation by Zeraḥyah ben Isaac Ben She'altiel Ḥen, MS Munich 111, fols. 1–83.

פ *Medical Aphorisms,* Hebrew translation by Nathan ha-Me'ati, MS Paris, Bibliothèque nationale, héb. 1173, (14th century), fols. 1–92.

Modern Editions

m Muntner, Süssman, ed., *Pirḳe Mosheh bi-refu'ah,* trans. Nathan ha-Me'ati.

r Rosner, Fred, trans., *The Medical Aphorisms of Moses Maimonides.*

Abbreviations

ed. Boudon	Galen, *Exhortation à l'etude de la medicine: Art médical,* ed. and trans. Véronique Boudon.
ed. de Lacy	*On the Doctrines of Hippocrates and Plato,* ed. and trans. Phillip de Lacy.
ed. Kühn	Galen, *Claudii Galeni opera omnia,* ed. C. G. Kühn.
*EI*²	*Encyclopedia of Islam.* New ed.
EJ	*Encyclopedia of Judaica.*
Galen, *De loc. aff.*	Arabic translation of Galen's *De locis affectis,* attributed to Ḥunayn. Ms. Wellcome Or. 14a, fols. 1–176.
Galen, *De usu part.*	Arabic translation of Galen's *De usu partium,* attributed to Ḥubaysh, revised by Ḥunayn. Ms. Paris 2853, fols. 1–301.
Galen, *In Hipp. De aere*	In Hippocratis *De aere aquis locis commentarius,* forthcoming edition and Arabic translation by G. Strohmaier.
Galen, *In Hipp. Epid. 1 & 2*	Galeni in *Hippocratis Epidemiarum libros I et II.* Ed. Ernst Wenkebach and Franz Pfaff.
Galen, *In Hipp. Epid. 3*	Galeni in *Hippocratis Epidemiarum librum III commentaria III.* Ed. Ernst Wenkebach.
Galen, *In Hipp. Epid. 6*	Galeni in *Hippocratis Epidemiarum librum VI commentaria I–VIII.* Ed. Ernst Wenkebach and Franz Pfaff.
trans. Brock	Galen, *On the Natural Faculties,* trans. Arthur John Brock.
trans. Deller	Deller, K. H., "Die Exzerpte des Moses Maimonides aus den Epidemienkommentaren des Galen."
trans. Goss	Galen, "On Movement of Muscles," trans. Charles Mayo Gross.
trans. Green	Galen, *A Translation of Galen's Hygiene,* trans. Robert Montraville Green.
trans. May	Galen, *On the Usefulness of the Parts of the Body,* trans. Margaret Tallmadge May.
trans. Savage-Smith	Galen, "Galen on Nerves, Veins, and Arteries," trans. Emilie Savage-Smith.
trans. Siegel	Galen, *Galen on the Affected Parts,* trans. Rudolph E. Siegel.

Other Symbols

< >	supplied by editor, in Arabic and Hebrew text
[ ]	supplied by translator, in English text
add.	added in
om.	omitted in
conj. Bos	editorial conjecture or correction
(!)	corrupt reading
(?)	doubtful reading

Transliteration and Citation Style

Transliterations from Arabic and Hebrew follow the romanization tables established by the American Library Association and the Library of Congress (*ALA-LC Romanization Tables: Transliteration Schemes for Non-Roman Scripts.* Compiled and edited by Randall K. Barry. Washington, D.C.: Library of Congress, 1997).

Passages from the *Aphorisms* are referenced by treatise and section number (e.g., 3.12). Maimonides' introduction is designated as treatise 0.

Foreword

Brigham Young University and its Middle Eastern Texts Initiative are pleased to sponsor and publish The Medical Works of Moses Maimonides. The texts that appear in this series are among the cultural treasures of the world, representing as they do the medieval efflorescence of Arabic-Islamic civilization—a civilization in which works of impressive intellectual stature were composed not only by Muslims but also by Christians, Jews, and others in a quest for knowledge that transcended religious and ethnic boundaries. Together they not only preserved the best of Greek thought but enhanced it, added to it, and built upon it a corpus of scientific and philosophical understanding that is properly the inheritance of all the peoples of the world.

As an institution of The Church of Jesus Christ of Latter-day Saints, Brigham Young University is honored to collaborate with Gerrit Bos and other members of the academic community in bringing this series to fruition, making these texts available to many for the first time. In doing so, we at the Middle Eastern Texts Initiative hope to serve our fellow human beings of all creeds and cultures. We also follow the admonition of our own religious tradition, to "seek . . . out of the best books words of wisdom," believing, indeed, that "the glory of God is intelligence."

—Daniel C. Peterson
D. Morgan Davis

Preface

The Medical Works of Moses Maimonides: Toward Critical Editions and Translations

It is a stunning and sad fact that, despite the unending accolades that Maimonides receives for his accomplishments in the field of philosophy, his surviving medical writings have still not received their scholarly due. Of his major works, three are available only in editions of the medieval Hebrew translations made from the Arabic in which these works were originally composed, and in modern translations based on the Hebrew—*Kitāb al-fuṣūl fī al-ṭibb* (Medical Aphorisms), *Sharḥ fuṣūl Abuqrāṭ* (Commentary on Hippocrates' Aphorisms), and *Kitāb al-sumūm wa al-taḥarruz min al-adwiya al-qattāla* (On Poisons and the Protection against Lethal Drugs). A fourth major work, *Mukhtaṣarāt li-kutub Jālīnūs* (Abridgements of the Works of Galen)—presumably the first medical work composed by Maimonides—survives only in part and has not been edited at all, though it is available in an incomplete English translation.

Unfortunately, the Hebrew editions of Maimonides' medical works as prepared by Süssman Muntner are unsatisfactory according to modern editorial standards, which demand a critical edition of the text based on all the available manuscripts, along with a critical apparatus. Equally unfortunately, the modern English translations by Fred Rosner, covering almost all of the medical writings by Maimonides, are flawed—not only because they are based on corrupt editions, but also because of many mistakes and misunderstandings of the Hebrew text. Although the Arabic editions of the treatises *On Hemorrhoids, On Coitus,* and *On the Regimen of Health,* all prepared by Hermann Kroner, are reliable in general, these also need to be revised, since it was often the case that Kroner had access to only a very limited number of manuscripts of a particular text.

Accordingly, the publication of critical editions and translations of the Arabic originals of these works is an urgent desideratum. It is only on the basis of such critical editions that scholarly research into Maimonides' medical works can and should proceed. These originals not only provide better readings than the often corrupt Hebrew translations, but they sometimes offer different versions and additions—as is the case, for instance, with the *Medical Aphorisms.* To deal with this situation, I set up a project in 1995—initially at University College, London, and sponsored by the Wellcome Trust, and now at the University of Cologne with the support of the Deutsche Forschungsgemeinschaft—to produce and publish critical editions of these vital works. The series is published through Brigham Young University's Middle Eastern Texts Initiative and includes the *Medical Aphorisms* (with extensive glossaries), *On Asthma, On Hemorrhoids,* and *On Poisons and the Protection against Lethal Drugs,* all edited and translated by Gerrit Bos with Latin translations edited by Michael McVaugh; *On Coitus,* edited and translated by Gerrit Bos with the Latin translation edited by Charles Burnett; *Commentary on Hippocrates' Aphorisms,* edited and translated by Carsten Schliwski; and *Abridgments of the Works of Galen,* and *The Regimen of Health.*

Acknowledgments

On this occasion I wish to thank Professor Daniel C. Peterson, editor-in-chief of the Middle Eastern Texts Initiative for his enthusiastic response to this project, and Dr. Glen M. Cooper for his many helpful suggestions regarding both content and form. I also thank Angela C. Barrionuevo, Alison Coutts, D. Morgan Davis, Dr. Muḥammad Eissa, Andrew Everett, and Sandra Thorne, for their dedicated editorial work. Thanks are due to Professor Vivian Nutton for his help in identifying Galenic sources, to Dr. Carsten Schliwski for his general assistance in the preparation of these volumes, and to David Wirmer for correcting the glossaries and indices. I am especially grateful to Kiki Peters for her commonsensical comments and corrections throughout the preparation of the different volumes of the series; and to Bibi, Boris, and Brendan—playing with them kept me healthy in body and mind.

Translator's Introduction

Moses Maimonides, known under his Arab name Abū ᶜImrān Mūsā ibn Maymūn ibn ᶜUbayd Allāh and his Jewish name Moshe ben Maimon, was not only one of the greatest philosophers and experts in Jewish law *(halakhah)*,[1] but an eminent physician as well. Born in Córdoba in 1138,[2] he was forced to leave his native city at an early age because of persecutions and the policy of religious intolerance adopted by the fanatical Muslim regime known as the Almohads.[3] After a sojourn of about twelve years in southern Spain, the family moved to Fez in the Maghreb. Some years later—probably around 1165—they moved again because of persecutions of the Jews in the Maghreb, this time going to Palestine. After a short sojourn of some months there, the family moved on to Egypt and settled in Fusṭāṭ, the ancient part of Cairo.

It was in Cairo that Maimonides started to practice and teach medicine, as well as pursue commercial activities in the India trade.[4] He became physician to al-Qāḍī al-Fāḍil, the famous counselor and secretary to Saladin.[5] Later, he became court physician to al-Malik al-Afḍal after the latter's ascension to the throne in the winter of 1198–99. It is generally assumed that Maimonides died in 1204. The theory that he served for some years as *nagid,* or leader, of the Jewish community in Egypt seems to be unfounded.[6]

Medical Works

Maimonides was a prolific author in the field of medicine, composing ten works considered authentic.[7] Of his major works in this field, the following are available only in editions of the medieval Hebrew translations and in modern language translations based on the Hebrew: *Sharḥ fuṣūl Abuqrāṭ* (Commentary on Hippocrates' Aphorisms),[8] *Kitāb al-sumūm wa al-taḥarruz min al-adwiya al-qattāla* (On Poisons and the Protection against Fatal Drugs),[9] and *Kitāb al-fuṣūl fī al-ṭibb* (Medical Aphorisms). A fourth major work, the *Mukhtaṣarāt li-kutub Jālīnūs* (Abridgements of the Works of Galen), survives only in part and has not been edited at all, but portions of it are available in an English translation.[10]

Of his smaller treatises, some have been edited. These include: *Kitāb fī al-jimāᶜ* (On Coitus);[11] *Fī tadbīr al-ṣiḥḥa* (On the Regimen of Health), written at the request of the Sultan al-Malik al-Afḍal;[12] *Maqāla fī bayān al-aᶜrāḍ wa-al-jawāb ᶜanhā* (On the Causes of Symptoms), probably written after 1198 for the same al-Malik al-Afḍal when his condition did not improve;[13] *Sharḥ asmāᵓ al-ᶜuqqār* (Commentary on the Names of Drugs);[14] *Risāla fī al-bawāsīr* (On Hemorrhoids);[15] and *Maqāla fī al-rabw* (On Asthma).[16]

Kitāb al-fuṣūl fī al-ṭibb (Medical Aphorisms)

Of Maimonides' medical works, the most famous and most voluminous is, without any doubt, the *Medical Aphorisms.* As a whole, it consists of twenty-five treatises comprised of approximately fifteen hundred aphorisms that are drawn for the most part from the works of Galen, covering every field of medicine. Its date of composition is uncertain. On the one hand, there are indications that Aphorisms numbers among the earlier medical works composed by Maimonides,[17] since it is quoted by him in his *Commentary on the Aphorisms of Hippocrates*[18] and since this latter work is mentioned by him in *On Asthma.*[19] On the other hand, a scribal note to MS Gotha 1937 seems to show that at least the twenty-fifth treatise was composed at the end of his life.[20] From this note, some scholars have concluded that the entire extant version of the *Medical Aphorisms* should be considered his last work.[21] Recently, Elinor Lieber has suggested that the first twenty-four treatises were composed at an early date and that the twenty-fifth treatise was composed at the end of Maimonides' life and added to the earlier treatises.[22] Internal evidence from the *Aphorisms* itself is possibly provided by aphorism 24.40. In this aphorism, Maimonides remarks that for a period of twenty years since his arrival in Egypt, he has observed twenty cases of diabetes. If one assumes that he arrived in Egypt around the year 1165, one might conclude that at least this section was written around 1185.

Of this work, the following sections have been published so far: (1) the introduction and six fragments;[23] (2) treatise 25, sections 57–68 (i.e., that part from treatise 25 that contains Maimonides' criticism of the philosophical doctrines to which Galen adhered);[24] and (3) treatise 25, sections 56–71.[25] The complete text is available in an edition of the medieval Hebrew translation prepared by Nathan ha-Me᾽ati between 1279 and 1283 in Rome[26] and in modern English translations.[27] Another medieval Hebrew translation prepared in 1277 by Zeraḥyah ben Isaac ben She᾽altiel Ḥen of Rome remains unedited.[28]

Each of the twenty-five treatises comprising the *Medical Aphorisms* deals with a subspecialty in medicine: The first three cover anatomy, physiology, and general pathology; 4 through 6, symptomatology; 7 through 14, etiology; 15, surgery; 16, gynecology; 17, hygiene; 18 through 20, diet; and 21 and 22, pharmacopoeia. Twenty-three provides explanations of obscure names and concepts in Galen's works; 24 is a collection of rare and interesting cases out of Galen's writings; and 25 offers criticism of Galen.[29] Most of the approximately fifteen hundred aphorisms in this work are based on the writings of Galen—whether they quote, paraphrase, or summarize his words—and some of them are no longer available in the original Greek. An example is the following: "As for laughter that occurs through the tickling of the armpits and the soles of the feet, as well as laughter that occurs when seeing or hearing comical things, it is impossible to isolate its cause."[30] This aphorism, a quotation from Galen's *De motibus manifestis et obscuris* (On Manifest and Hidden Movements), survives only in a Latin translation by Niccolò da Reggio[31] and an Arabic translation that I am currently editing. Muntner assumed erroneously that the Hebrew translation of Galen's *De motibus,* entitled *Ba-tenuᶜot ha-mukhraḥot,* is identical with Galen's Περὶ θώρακος καὶ πνεύμονος κινήσεως (On the Movement of the Chest and Lung). This assumption was adopted by Rosner as well.

Other quotations which have not survived in any other source are, for instance, treatise 16.1, 3, 9, 14–16, 20, 30, and 35. These derive from Galen's lost commentary on Hippocrates' *De mulierum affectibus* (Diseases of Women). However, the authenticity of this work is uncertain; it is not mentioned by Ḥunayn ibn Isḥāq, but only by Ibn Abī Uṣaybiᶜa.[32] Another work of doubtful authenticity quoted by Maimonides is the one entitled *On the Signs of Death.* Maimonides states:

> Concerning chronic illnesses such as orthopnea, stones, tumors in the nose, bad ulcers, and the like, most of these afflictions occurring in youngsters and children are cured in forty days or seven months or seven years. Some of them [are cured] before the pubic hair starts to grow and, in the case of girls, at the time of menstruation. *De signis mortis.*[33]

This work does not appear in the lists of works composed by Galen or ascribed to him.[34] The Arabic tradition has preserved a number of texts under this title that are ascribed to Hippocrates, all in manuscript, whose central subject is the signs of death as derived from the efflorescences of the skin. A text under this title ascribed to the famous philosopher and physician al-Kindī is actually an adaptation of a part of Hippocrates' *Prognostica* (Prognostics).[35] In one case, the *Medical Aphorisms*—that is, the Arabic tradition quoted by Maimonides—has preserved a better reading based on a lost Greek manuscript. The following quotation from Galen's *De usu partium* 9 is an example:

> Arteries and veins in the whole body are connected with all the parts that [need] connection [with them]. They are near one another and sometimes so close together that the veins are in contact with the arteries. Thus, one always finds the veins directly upon the arteries, *with the sole exception of the brain;* for the arteries ascend to it from below to facilitate the upward movement of the pneuma, while the veins descend to the brain from the crown of the head to facilitate the transport of food to the brain.[36]

As to the section missing in the Greek text, Margaret May, the translator of this text, remarks in a penetrating analysis:

> It is the difference between the modes of insertion of the veins and arteries into the encephalon and into the other parts to which attention is being called here, and we should therefore expect that "in none of these parts does the vein come to its insertion from above and the artery from below [as they do in the encephalon]." There is no indication, however, of any variation in the manuscripts, so that we are left wondering how the transposition came to be made.[37]

Other aphorisms are recorded partly in Galen's words and partly in those of Maimonides. Still other aphorisms are completely reformulated by Maimonides, as he explicitly states in the introduction:

> I don't claim to have authored these aphorisms. . . . I rather say that I have selected them; that is, I have collected them from what Galen said in his books, both what he said in his own treatises and what he said in his commentaries to Hippocrates.
>
> I have not been as fastidious with regard to these aphorisms as I was in my epitomes, where I quoted Galen's very words, as I stipulated in the introduction to the epitomes. . . . Instead, some of the aphorisms that I have selected are the very words of Galen, or his and those of

> Hippocrates, since the two of them are combined in Galen's commentaries to Hippocrates' writings; for others, the aphorism is partly Galen's words and partly my own; and for yet other aphorisms, it is my own words that express the idea that Galen mentioned.[38]

An important element of the reformulation process is abbreviation. Take, for example, aphorism 23.66, which is derived from Galen's *De locis affectis* (On the Affected Parts of the Body), in its Arabic translation by Ḥunayn ibn Isḥāq.[39] When one compares Ḥunayn's translation with that of Maimonides,[40] it becomes clear that the latter has summarized and abbreviated nonessential parts of this text:[41]

Maimonides:

العلّة التي يسمّيها الأطبّاء البيضة والخوذة هو مرض من أمراض الرأس وهو صداع مزمن عسر الانقلاع يصير بالأسباب اليسيرة إلى أن ينوب نوائب عظيمة حتّى أنّ صاحبه لا يحتمل صوت كلام ولا ضوءا ساطعا ولا حركة وأحبّ الأشياء إليه الاستلقاء في الظلمة لعظم الوجع

> al-ᶜillatu allatī yusammīhā al-aṭibbāᵓu al-bayḍata wa-al-khūdhata huwa maraḍun min amrāḍi al-raᵓsi wa-huwa ṣudāᶜun muzminun ᶜasiru al-inqilāᶜi yaṣīru bi-al-asbābi al-yasīrati ilā an yanūba nawāᵓiba ᶜaẓīmatan ḥattā anna ṣāḥibahu la yaḥtimilu ṣauta kalāmin wa-lā ḍawᵓan sāṭiᶜan wa-lā ḥarakatan wa-aḥabbu al-ashyāᵓi ilayhi al-istilqāᵓu fī al-ẓulmati li-ᶜaẓmi al-wajᶜi.

> "The disease called *al-bayḍa wa-al-khūdha* by the physicians is a disease affecting the head. It is a chronic headache which is difficult to eliminate. It flares up due to minor stimuli, [causing] such severe paroxysms that the patient cannot bear the sound of speaking, nor bright light, nor any movement. He would like most of all to lie down in the dark because of the severity of the pain."

Ḥunayn:

العلّة التي يسمّيها الأطبّاء البيضة والخوذة ما من أحد يشكّ فيها ولا يرتاب بها فيقول إنّها ليست مرض من أمراض الرأس وذلك أنّ هذه العلّة في المثل إذا وصفه إنسان وحصّلها بكلام وجيز قال إنّها صداع مزمن عسر الانقلاع يصير بالأسباب اليسيرة إلى أن ينوب نوائب عظيمة جدّا حتّى أنّ صاحبه لا يقدر أن يحتمل صوت شيئ يقرع ولا صوت كلام له فضل شدّة ولا ضوءا ساطعا ولا حركة لكنّه يكون أحبّ الأشياء إليه أن يبقى مستلقيا في الظلمة لعظم الوجع

> al-ᶜillatu allatī yusammīhā al-aṭibbāᵓu al-bayḍata wa-al-khūdhata *mā min aḥadin yashukku fīhā wa-lā yartābu bihā fa-yaqūlu innahā laysat* maraḍan min amrāḍi al-raᵓsi *wa-dhālika anna hādhihi al-ᶜillata fī al-mathal idhā waṣafaha insānun wa-ḥaṣṣalaha bi-kalāmin wajīzin qāla innahā* ṣudāᶜun muzminun ᶜasiru al-inqilāᶜi yaṣīru bi-al-asbābi al-yasīrati ilā an yanūba nawāᵓiba aẓīmatan *jiddan* ḥattā anna ṣāḥibahu la *yaqdaru an* yaḥtimila ṣauta *shayᵓin yuqraᶜu wa-lā ṣauta* kalāmin *lahu faḍlu shiddatin* wa-lā ḍawᵓan sāṭiᶜan wa-lā ḥarakatan *lākinnahu yakūnu* aḥabbu al-ashyāᵓi ilayhi *an yabqā* mustilqiᵓan fī al-ẓulmati li-ᶜaẓmi al-wajᶜi.

> "*Concerning* the disease called *al-bayḍa wa-al-khūdha* by the physicians, *no one has any doubts or misgivings such that he would say that it is not* a disease affecting the head. *For, if someone were to characterize and describe this disease in a concise way, he would say that* it is a chronic headache that is difficult to eliminate and that flares up due to minor stimuli, [causing] such [*very*] severe paroxysms that the patient cannot bear *the sound made by something, nor* the sound of *extremely loud* speaking, nor bright light, nor any movement. *But* he would like most of all to remain in a prone position in the dark because of the severity of the pain."

In yet other cases, Maimonides adds certain elements to the text, probably since these are essential, in his view, for a correct interpretation of the text. Note, for instance, aphorism 3.73, taken from Galen, *De sanitate tuenda* 6.5–6:

> If you find that someone falls ill only on rare occasions, do not change any of his habits in his whole way of life. But if someone falls ill frequently, you should look for its cause and eliminate it. *It is beyond doubt that this [occurs] through a change in one or more of his habits. You should also consider concerning someone whose habit you want to change whether or not such a change can be well tolerated by him. De Sanitate Tuenda* [1].[42]

In aphorism 1.62, Maimonides correctly adds to Galen's theory that the right kidney lies higher than the left kidney the fact that this is true for some living beings only. May suggests that Galen "was almost certainly describing conditions in some species of ape."[43]

Maimonides is, as Schacht and Meyerhof remark, "an excellent guide through the basic ideas of Galen for students of the history of medicine."[44] However, Maimonides also refers to many famous Arab physicians, such as Ḥunayn ibn Isḥāq, Ibn Sīnā, and al-Rāzī. And again, many of these quotations come from lost or unedited works.[45] Unlike most of his colleagues, Maimonides provides (usually correct) general references to the sources he quotes.[46] He proves himself to be an independent and critical physician who tries to eradicate prejudices and dictated dogmas in medicine, even if they originate with a physician as famous as Galen. For instance, in aphorism 1.34 he criticizes Galen for not having solved the question of how the will of someone who is asleep or absent-minded can be nullified while he yet carries out voluntary movements. His systematic criticism of Galen in medical and philosophical issues forms the subject of the twenty-fifth treatise, in which Maimonides charges Galen with more than forty contradictions in his work and with ignorance in philosophical matters.

Maimonides' *Medical Aphorisms* enjoyed great popularity in medieval western Europe. In the thirteenth century it was translated into Latin. Of this translation, at least two different versions are extant in many editions. One of them, from the hand of John of Capua, was published as an incunabulum, first in Bologna in 1489 and again in Venice in 1497, and was rapidly followed by numerous Latin editions.[47] From the eleventh until the fifteenth century the Aphorisms was, as Muntner remarks, "the most widely known and wanted repetitorium of Galen."[48] It was quoted and recommended as a medical textbook by Jean de Touremire, professor of medicine in Montpellier (d. 1396); he referred to it as *Flores Galieni.* The fourteenth-century French surgeon Guy de Chauliac refers to it repeatedly in his *Inventarium sive Chirurgia Magna,* which he completed in 1363.[49]

In Jewish circles, it became influential through the two Hebrew translations mentioned above. Both translations were very popular and often copied by Jewish scribes. Nathan's translation is extant in not less than twenty-three manuscripts, seventeen of them written in Spanish or Provençal script, which means that they were mostly distributed in Spain and France. Zeraḥyah's translation is extant in fifteen manuscripts and was only copied in non-Sephardic scripts, ten of which were in Italian script. This means that his translation was mostly distributed in Italy.[50] This limited distribution may be explained from the fact that Zeraḥyah's translation contains many terms in Italian. In a letter to his friend Isaac—the pope's physician, more widely known as Master Gaio—the prominent Italian Jewish philosopher Hillel ben Samuel of Verona (ca. 1220–1295) requested copies of Nathan ha-Me᾿ati's Hebrew translations of both the *Medical Aphorisms* and the *Commentary on Hippocrates' Aphorisms.* Hillel instructed Isaac to have a scribe copy them regardless of the price, since he loved these books so much.[51] The Jewish philosopher Shem Tov ben

Joseph ibn Falaquera quotes from treatise 25.59, 69–71 in his *Moreh ha-moreh,* a commentary on Maimonides' *Dalālat al-ḥāʾirīn* (Guide of the Perplexed), which he completed around the year 1280.[52] Moshe Narboni (ca. 1300–1365) frequently draws upon the *Medical Aphorisms* in his *Sefer oraḥ ḥayyim.* An example is the following magical remedy for hard abscesses: "If you bring the marcasite stone[53] to a red-hot glow with fire and sprinkle vinegar on that and place the limb that has a hard abscess above the vapour that rises from it, you will observe something amazing from its dissolution as if it were an act of magic."[54] Narboni notes that "Rabbeinu Mosheh related this in his *Sefer ha-moreh* (Moreh nevukhim) and explained it by quoting the Sages' dictum: 'whatever is used as a remedy is not [forbidden] on account of the ways of the Amorite.' "[55] A comparison of Narboni's quotation with the Hebrew translation of the *Aphorisms* prepared by Nathan ha-Meʾati (ed. Muntner) and with that of Zeraḥyah ben Isaac ben Sheʾaltiel Ḥen shows clearly that Narboni has consulted Nathan's text.

Moshe Narboni:

אבן מרקשיטא כשתלובן באש ויזו עליה חומץ ותושם <על> האבר שיש בו מורסא קשה על האיד העולה ממנו תראה בהתכתה דבר מופלא כאלו הוא מפעולות הכשפים

Even markashiṭa ke-she-telubban ba-esh ṿe-yazzu ᶜaleiha ḥomets ṿe-tusam (ᶜal) ha-ever she-yesh bo mursa ḳashah ᶜal ha-eid ha-ᶜoleh mimmennu tirʾeh be-hat-takhatah davar mufla ke-illu hu mi-peᶜullot ha-keshafim.

Nathan ha-Meʾati:

אבן מרקשיתא כשתלובן באש ויוזה עליו חומץ ותושם <על> האבר שיש בו מורסא קשה על האיד העולה ממנו תראה בהתכתה דבר מופלא כאלו הוא מפעולות הכשפים

Even markashita ke-she-telubban ba-esh ṿe-yuzzeh ᶜalaṿ ḥomets ṿe-tusam (ᶜal) ha-ever she-yesh bo mursa ḳashah ᶜal ha-eid ha-ᶜoleh mimmennu tirʾeh be-hat-takhatah davar mufla ke-illu hu mi-peᶜullot ha-keshafim.

Zeraḥyah:

אבן המרקשיתא כשתלבנהו באור ותזה עליו חומץ והושם האבר אשר בו מורסה קשה על העשן העולה ממנו תראה בהתרתו פלאות וכאילו הוא פעולת הכשפות

> *Even ha-markashita ke-she-telabbenehu ba-ur ve-tazzeh ʿalav ḥomets ve-husam ha-ever asher bo mursah kashah ʿal he-ʿashan ha-ʿoleh mimmennu tirʾeh be-hattarato pelaʾot u-khe-illu hu peʿullat ha-keshafot.*

In an anonymous compilation on fevers, written in old French in Hebrew script and probably dating from the thirteenth century, the author remarks that he wants to translate everything from the "Pirḳe Rabbenu Mosheh" concerning the crisis of fevers.[56] And a recipe for quartan fever found in *Medical Aphorisms* 10.56 and derived from Galen's *De theriaca ad pisonem* is quoted by Salmias (Salamias) of Lunel in a treatise on fevers in the name of Maimonides.[57] Gerson Ben Ezechias of Beaumes (b. ca. 1373), the author of a medical handbook in rhyme, remarks that he had read in the presence of the *nasi* Todros of Narbonne or his son Kalonymos a variety of medical treatises, among which were the "chapters of Moses."[58] A gloss that appears in the *Sefer ha-ḳibbusin,* a treatise on purgatives translated from the Latin, gives a recipe for headaches derived from the "Pirḳe Mosheh."[59] Rabbi Solomon Ben Abraham ha-Kohen who lived in sixteenth-century Greece quotes in his *Responsa* aphorism 16.18, which is the case of a woman who suffered from hysterical suffocation and who through touching her genitals when she inserted medicines into her womb had an experience similar to an orgasm and then discharged a thick clot of semen and thus found relief from her afflictions.[60] The popularity of the *Medical Aphorisms* in Jewish circles confirms Lawrence Conrad's suggestion that "the Greek medical corpus was mediated to physicians of the Jewish communities primarily as extracts and easily learned statements, rather than through the fundamental works where medical theory and practice were worked out in detail."[61] In the introduction to the *Aphorisms,* Maimonides explicitly states that he wants to use the format of aphorisms in order to present them in a manner that could be clearly understood and yet easily memorized. In the West, twelfth-century teachers of medicine preferred works with a schematic or aphoristic presentation, such as the *Articella,* whose popularity persisted in Montpellier itself well beyond the thirteenth century.[62]

In short, *Medical Aphorisms* enriches our knowledge of Maimonides' activity as a physician, the transmission of classical Greek learning to both Europe and the Middle East, medieval Hebrew and Latin translation techniques, the medieval reaction to Galen, the interplay of medicine and philosophy, and the cosmopolitan character of medieval Islamic medicine.

Muntner's Edition of the Hebrew Translation and Rosner's English Translation

Muntner's edition (**m**) of Nathan ha-Me᾿ati's Hebrew translation is, unfortunately, eclectic in its approach; though primarily based, as the editor remarks in the introduction, on MS Paris 1173 (**פ**),[63] it lacks a critical apparatus specifying precisely which manuscript or manuscript tradition of Nathan ha-Me᾿ati's translation was consulted at any given point in the edition. Moreover, it is replete with errors and therefore unreliable.[64]

More unfortunate still, Muntner's Hebrew edition was the basis for the first English translation prepared by Muntner and Rosner in 1970 (Rosner and Muntner, ed. and trans., *Medical Aphorisms of Moses Maimonides*). Consequently, the well-known historian of Islamic medicine, Manfred Ullmann, was forced to conclude that "[this translation] contains innumerable misunderstandings and errors, which could have been avoided had the original Arabic text been used."[65] Yet another fault of this translation is that Rosner reads modern ideas into the medical theories expounded and often presents these in a modern medical terminology inappropriate to the humoralist theory that was fundamental to ancient and medieval medicine.[66]

Acknowledging this criticism of their translation, Rosner undertook a second revised translation on his own, which was published in 1989 (**r**). But this translation, too, suffers from many mistakes and corruptions, since it is still based on the noncritical and inaccurate edition of Muntner. Instead of this edition, Rosner should have consulted the Arabic original more consistently. Moreover, many mistakes could have been avoided if he had used, in addition to the Hebrew translation by Nathan ha-Me᾿ati, the one prepared by Zeraḥyah ben Isaac ben She᾿altiel Ḥen, for in several cases Rosner's mistakes originate from errors or lack of clarity in Nathan's translation. The list of translation errors from Muntner's and Rosner's editions featuring in the supplement to this edition may substantiate this claim. It should be noted that this list is not exhaustive but is, rather, a selection of the most striking examples, resulting from a comparison of Rosner's English translation (**r**), Muntner's edition (**m**) of the Hebrew translation by Nathan ha-Me᾿ati (**פ**),[67] and Zeraḥyah's Hebrew translation[68] (**ב** and **מ**) with the Arabic text of ms. Gotha (**G**). The question of whether Nathan ha-Me᾿ati was a poor translator in comparison to Zeraḥyah cannot be answered unequivocally on the basis of this limited research, since it is possible that the Arabic manuscript(s) he consulted was (were) of an inferior quality and that the surviving Hebrew manuscripts containing his translation have been corrupted to a certain degree by scribes. Moreover, scholars have yet to critically evaluate the translation activity of medieval Jewish scholars in the field of medicine. Further information on the different methods of translation they used can be drawn from the forthcoming glossary to the aphorisms, which gives a comparative list of technical terms drawn from Maimonides' Arabic text and from both Hebrew translations.[69] One striking difference between the two Hebrew translators is that Zeraḥyah regularly employs equivalents in Romance languages, unlike Nathan.[70] In order to facilitate the consultation of the Hebrew material there will be separate alphabetical indices of both Nathan's and Zeraḥyah's Hebrew terminology. These indices can serve as an important tool for identifying the authorship of anonymous translations of medical material[71] and for the insertion of medical terminology into the dictionaries of the Hebrew language.

Manuscripts of the *Kitāb al-fuṣūl fī al-ṭibb* (Medical Aphorisms)

The *Kitāb al-fuṣūl fī al-ṭibb* is known to be extant in the following manuscripts:

(1) Gotha 1937 (**G**); fols. 6–273 (fol. 7 numbered twice); Naskh script.[72] A considerable section of the text, from treatise 6.10 beginning at *al-mawt* to treatise 7.16 ending at *min amthāl,* is missing.[73] According to the colophon on fol. 273a that appears after Aphorism 25.55, the scribe copied the text from a copy of the original redaction of the work by Maimonides' nephew Abū al-Maʾālī (or al-Maʾānī) ibn Yūsuf ibn ʿAbdallāh.[74] The scribe adds that he found a note in the text in which Abū al-Maʾālī remarks that in the case of the first twenty-four *maqālāt,* Maimonides would correct his autograph notes and that he, Abū al-Maʾālī, would then make a fair copy and correct it in Maimonides' presence, but that the text of the twenty-fifth *maqāla* was copied by him in the beginning of the year 602 A.H. (August 1205), after the death of Maimonides, so the latter had not been able to do the redaction.[75] Although it is generally agreed that this manuscript has preserved the best readings,[76] it should be noted that in some cases the text suffers from a certain carelessness by the scribe, resulting in mistakes and corruptions. Moreover, the language he employs is sometimes extremely vulgar and colloquial.

(2) Leiden 1344, Or. 128, 1 (**L**); fols. 1–140; Maghribī script.[77] The manuscript ends on fol. 140b with the following colophon:

> This is the end of the treatise—praise be to God—and the completion of the *Book of Aphorisms* of the most perfect and unique scholar Mūsā ibn Maymūn ibn ᶜUbaydallāh, the Israelite, from Cordova—may God be pleased with him. The copying [of the text] was completed in the month of May of the year 1362, according to the calendar of al-Ṣufr, in the city of Ṭulayṭula—may God protect it—and it was written by Yūsuf ibn Isḥāq ibn Shabbathay, the Israelite.

The calendar of al-Ṣufr was common in Spain, especially among Christians, and started about thirty-eight years before the Christian calendar.[78] Accordingly, the manuscript was written in May 1324 in Toledo. More than any of the other manuscripts, the language of this manuscript conforms to the rules of classical Arabic; the influence of vulgarization is thus far less pronounced than in the others.

(3) Paris BN, héb. 1210 (**P**); fols. 1–130; Judaeo-Arabic; no date.[79] The manuscript contains only treatises 1–9 (the last one incomplete), part of treatise 24, and the major part of treatise 25. According to the inscription on fol. 1v, the manuscript was once in the possession of Rabbi Meir ha-QNZ(?)Y. The text has been copied carefully, so that there are only a few mistakes; the top section has been stained to the degree that the first lines are hard to read.

(4) Escorial, Real Biblioteca de El Escorial 868 (**E**); fols. 117–26 (numbered in reverse order); Maghribī script.[80] According to the colophon, this text was copied in the city of Qalᶜa by Mūsā ibn Sūshān al-Yahūdī in the year 1380 (read 1388), corresponding to the year 5149 since the creation. The text offers a close parallel to manuscript **L**, both having many otherwise unique readings in common, including whole paragraphs not appearing in any other manuscript—as, for instance, treatise 3.52.

(5) Escorial, Real Biblioteca de El Escorial 869 (**S**); fols. 176–1(numbered in reverse order), Oriental script; no date.[81] The text, missing an important section between treatises 10.27 and 21.73, finishes at treatise 25.58. The text of this manuscript is closely related to **G**.

(6) Oxford, Bodleian, Uri 412, Poc. 319, cat. Neubauer 2113 (**B**); fols. 1–123; Judaeo-Arabic; Sephardic semicursive script.[82] According to the colophon, the text was copied by Makhluf ben Rabbi Shmuᵓel he-Ḥazan DMNSY (from Le Mans?) and completed on the eleventh of Elul 5112 (1352 C.E.).[83] Numerous Hebrew versions derived from the Hebrew translation prepared by Nathan ha-Meᵓati have been added to the text above

the lines and in the margins. The text suffers from many omissions and corruptions but does provide some unique variant readings—as, for instance, treatise 3.22: اللحم المركب; a unique, correct version according to Galen's τῆς συνθήτου σαρκὸς.[84]

(7) Oxford, Bodleian, Hunt. Donat 33, Uri 423, cat. Neubauer 2114 (**O**); 78 fols.; Sephardic semicursive script; ca. 1300(?).[85] The text begins with treatise 23, continues with the end of treatise 6 to treatise 24 (incomplete), and ends with treatise 12. Besides, it contains two sections from the third treatise of *Medical Aphorisms:* 3.59, beginning with من العفونة until 3.84: الصداع الشديد, and 3.89, beginning with بحسب until 3.98: تغيّرا.

(8) Oxford, Bodleian, Hunt. 356, Uri 426, cat. Neubauer 2115; 107 fols., Oriental semicursive script; late thirteenth century.[86] The text runs from treatise 10 (but not from its beginning) to treatise 24 (but not to its end).

(9) Göttingen 99. This manuscript was copied by Antonius Deussingius in the year 1635 in Leiden from **L.**[87]

(10) Istanbul Velieddin 2525.[88]

For this edition of Maimonides' *Medical Aphorisms 1–5,* the following manuscripts have been consulted: Gotha 1937 (**G**), Leiden 1344 (**L**), Paris 1210 (**P**), Escorial 868 (**E**) and 869 (**S**), and Oxford 2113 (**B**). These manuscripts can be divided into two main groups: **S** and **G**; and **E**, **L**, **B**, and **P**. This second main group can be subdivided into two subgroups: **E** and **L**, and **B** and **P**. This edition is based mainly on **G**.

The text of Maimonides' *Medical Aphorisms* has been edited in Arabic rather than in Hebrew characters because scholars today consider it likely that Maimonides composed his medical writings in Arabic script. Meyerhof remarks that "Maimonides composed all his medical writings in Arabic, probably using Arabic characters, as he had nothing to hide from the Muslims."[89] Blau suggests that "[a Jewish] author, when addressing himself to the general public, including Muslims and Christians ([as is the case] in medical writings . . .), might have used Arabic script, but when addressing a Jewish audience wrote in Hebrew characters."[90] According to S. M. Stern, "All of Maimonides' medical works were naturally published in Arabic script, since otherwise they would have been of no use to the non-Jewish public," although he adds that "Maimonides drafted in Hebrew script books ultimately to be published in Arabic script" because "writing in Hebrew script came to him more easily and more naturally."[91] Langermann, on the other hand, asserts that "it seems likely that . . . many of Maimonides' medical writings" were "originally [written] . . . in Arabic characters, and . . . only afterwards . . . transcribed into Hebrew characters."[92]

In editing the Arabic text, which is written in the Middle Arabic typical for this genre, I have adhered to the guidelines formulated by Oliver Kahl. Morphological and syntactical errors and even grievous offenses against the grammar of classical Arabic have neither been included in the apparatus nor changed or corrected at all. Nor have peculiarities of orthography been included in the critical apparatus. They have either been spelled in the conventional way or allowed to remain in their original forms, as the need for clarity dictated.[93] In some cases I have corrected Maimonides' Arabic version on the basis of corresponding Arabic translations of the Galenic treatises he quotes.

MEDICAL APHORISMS

TREATISES 1–5

◆

The Book of Medical Aphorisms

composed by Mūsā ibn ᶜUbayd Allāh al-Qurṭubī al-Isrāᵓīlī

◆

In the name of God, the Merciful, the Compassionate
O Lord, make [our task] easy

[Author's Introduction]

Says Mūsā ibn ᶜUbayd Allāh, the Israelite, from Córdoba: People have often composed works in the form of aphorisms on [different] kinds of sciences. The science most in need of this is the science of medicine, because it has branches of knowledge that are difficult to conceptualize, like most of the exact sciences,[1] and [because] it has branches of knowledge that are difficult only with respect to remembering what has been written down about them, just like the knowledge of one of the perfect languages.[2] As for the science of medicine, its conceptualization and the understanding of its concepts are not as difficult as in [the case] of the exact sciences. However, aspiring [to master] this science is difficult in most cases because it requires retaining a very large amount of memorized material,[3] not merely of general principles but also [of] particulars, which can almost be compared to the individual details that cannot be encompassed by the knowledge of one individual scholar, as one can demonstrate for himself.

كتاب الفصول في الطبّ

تأليف موسى ابن ميمون ابن عبيد اللّه القرطبي الإسرائيلي

بسم اللّه الرحمن الرحيم ربّ يسّر

قال موسى بن عبيد اللّه القرطبي الإسرائيلي: كثيرا ما ألّف الناس تواليف على طريق الفصول في أنواع من العلوم وأحوج العلوم في ذلك علم الطبّ وذلك أنّ ثمّ معارف تعسر من جهة تصوّرها كأكثر التعاليم وثمّ معارف تعسر من جهة حفظ ما دوّن فيها لا غير كمعرفة علم لغة من اللغات الكاملة. وأمّا علم الطبّ فإنّه ليس تصوّره ولا فهم معانيه بالعسر كالتعاليم وإنّما يصعب مرام هذا العلم في أكثر الحالات من كونه يحتاج إلى محفوظ كثير جدّا لا حفظ الكلّيات فقط بل وحفظ جزئيات تكاد أن تقرب من الشخصيات التي لا يحيط بها علم عالم من البشر كما قد تبرهن.

١–٢ كتاب الفصول . . . الإسرائيلي] om. ESLP : فصول موسى القرطبي في الطبّ B || ٣ بسم اللّه . . . ربّ يسّر] بسم اللّه الرحمن الرحيم S : بسم اللّه الرحمن الرحي والحمد للّه ربّ العالمين L : ربّ يسّر P : رضي اللّه عنه B : بسم اللّه الرحمن الرحيم عليه توكّلت وبه وحده استعين لا ربّ سواه ‹ . . . › E || ٤ قال] الحكيم الفاضل الفيلسوف الأكمل الأوحد العلّامة add. L | بن] ميمون add. G[1] || ٥ في ذلك] لذلك BP : إلى EL || ٧–٨ فإنّه . . . بالعسر] فإنّه لا يعصر تصوّره ولا فهم معانيه L || ٨ كونه] جهة ما E || ١٠ تبرهن] يتبرهن B

These works composed in the form of aphorisms are undoubtedly easy to retain; they help their reader to understand and retain their objectives. Therefore, the most eminent of the physicians, Hippocrates, has written his famous work in the form of aphorisms.[4] Later on, many physicians followed his example and composed aphorisms, such as the *Aphorisms* of the famous al-Rāzī,[5] the *Aphorisms* of al-Sūsī,[6] the *Aphorisms* of Ibn Māsawayh,[7] and others.

It is clear to everyone who pays even the slightest attention that everyone who has composed aphorisms in any field of science did not compose them with the intention that those aphorisms would be sufficient for that science or that they would encompass all its principles. But one who has composed aphorisms according to this method has done so concerning matters he thought should always be retained, or [thought to be] neglected, or [thought] would be beneficial for [describing] that which one needs in most cases. In short, the intention of one who has composed aphorisms has not been to encompass everything that one needs in the field of that science—neither Hippocrates in his *Aphorisms* nor Abū Naṣr al-Fārābī[8] in anything he composed in the way of aphorisms, let alone others.

I have made these preliminary remarks merely as a justification for those aphorisms that I have included in my book. And I do not claim to have authored these aphorisms that I have set down in writing. I would rather say that I have selected them—that is, I have selected them from Galen's words from all his books, both from his original works and from his commentaries to the books of Hippocrates. In these aphorisms I have not adhered to the method that I followed in the *Epitomes,* in which I quoted Galen's very words, as I stipulated in the introduction to the *Epitomes.* Rather, most of the aphorisms that I have selected are in the very words of Galen, or in his words and the words of Hippocrates, because the words

وهـــذه التواليف التي تؤلّف على طريق الفصول ســـهلة الحفظ بلا شـــكّ معينة لقارئها على فهم أغراضها وحفظها ولذلك ألّف فاضل الأطبّاء بقراط كتابه المشـــهور مفصّلا. وقد ألّف بعده كثير من الأطبّاء مقتفيا لأثره فصولا كفصول الرازي المشـــهور وفصول السوسي وفصول ابن ماسويه وغيرهم.

وممّا يبين لكلّ واحد من الناظرين بأيســـر تأمّل أنّ كلّ من ألّف فصولا في علم ما لـــم يؤلّفها على أنّ تلك الفصـــول كافية في ذلك العلم أو محيطة بجملة أصوله. وإنّما ألّـــف كلّ من ألّف على هذه الطريقة فصولا في معـــان رأى أنّ تلك المعاني يجب أن تكون محفوظة دائما أو أنّ تلك المعاني مغفولا عنها أو أنّ تلك المعاني تفيد معظم ما يحتاج إليه. وبالجملة أنّ الغرض الذي قصده كلّ من قيّد فصولا لم يكن الإحاطة بكلّ ما يحتاج إليه في ذلك العلم لا ابقراط في فصوله ولا أبو نصر الفارابي في كلّ ما ألّفه على جهة الفصول وناهيك من سواهما.

وإنّمـــا قدّمت ما قدّمته اعتـــذارا عن هذه الفصول التـــي ضمّنتها كتابي هذا. وهـــذه الفصول التي أثبتّها لا أقول ألّفتها بل أقول اخترتها وذلك أنّي التقطتها من كلام جالينوس من جميع كتبه أعني من كلامه الذي أتى به على جهة التأليف ومن كلامه في شروحه لكتب ابقراط. ولم التزم في هذه الفصول ما التزمته في المختصرات من كونـــي أتيت فيها بنصّ كلام جالينوس كما اشـــترطت في صدر المختصرات بل هذه الفصول التي اخترتها أكثرها هو نصّ كلام جالينوس أو كلامه وكلام ابقراط لاختلاط

---

٢ وحفظهـــا] om. E | بقـــراط] ابقـــراط P || ٣ بعـــده] أيضـــا add. B | كثير] أيضا add. EP | لأثره] لأمره SG : لآثاره E | المشـــهور] المشـــهورة P || ٥ يبين] يتبين B | واحد] أحد BP || ٩ مـــن] واحـــد E || ١٠ ابقـــراط] بقراط SB || ١٢ وإنّما] واما (!)B || ١٣ أثبتّها] ضمنتهـــا E || ١٥ ابقـــراط] بقـــراط S || ١٦ أتيت فيها بنـــصّ] أثيت فيها نصّ (!)B || ١٦–١٧ كمـــا . . . نـــصّ كلام جالينـــوس] om. B || ١٧ أكثرهـــا] om. L | هـــو] om. S : هي L | ابقراط] بقراط SB

of both are mixed in Galen's commentaries to Hippocrates' books; [in the case of] others, the sense [expressed] in the aphorism is partly in Galen's words and partly in my own; [in the case of] yet other aphorisms, my own words express the idea that Galen mentioned.[9] What has prompted me to do so is the fact that the idea of that aphorism becomes clear only [after reading] from scattered places in Galen's lengthy exposition. I have gathered the sum of the idea of that aphorism and have articulated it in a concise expression. Since I know that there are more people who blindly follow the opinion of someone else than people who investigate for themselves and that there are more deficient [people] than learned people, I considered it appropriate to refer, at the end of every aphorism I cite, to that section in Galen's exposition in which he has explained that aphorism. So, if someone has doubts about the wording of that aphorism or about the idea expressed in it, he can easily look up that section and find that aphorism—whether he finds it in Galen's very words, or mostly so, or [whether] he finds that idea without omission or addition in Galen's exposition in that section, even if it is expressed in different words—so that his doubts are dispelled.

No one should protest to me that, while I know that this aphorism is mentioned by Galen in a certain section, its idea is also referred to by him in another section, or that he has repeated it in a number of places; for, if I were to refer [the reader] to one of these [other] places, the same objection would still apply. To refer to all the places is superfluous and has no use at all; it is, rather, a multiplication of words. But I preferred [to quote] his expression of an idea that is often repeated in his exposition in [only] one of its places and have recorded it [in that way]. Nor should one protest to me and say: "How could you write down an aphorism

قوليهما في شــروح جالينوس لكتب بقراط. وبعضها يكون بعض معنى ذلك الفصل بنــصّ كلام جالينوس وبعضه من كلامي وبعض فصول منها هي من كلامي عبارة عن ذلــك المعنى الذي ذكره جالينوس. والذي دعاني إلى ذلك كون معنى ذلك الفصل لم يتبيّن إلا من مواضع متفرّقة في طيّ كلام كثير لجالينوس. فالتقطت جملة معنى ذلك الفصل وعبّرت عنه بعبارة وجيزة. ولعلمي بكون المقلّدين من الناس أكثر من الناظرين والاشرار أكثر من الاخيار رأيت أن أنبّه في آخر كلّ فصل آتي به على المقالة من كلام جالينــوس التي بيّن فيها ذلك الفصل. فــإذا اتّهم أحد نصّ كلام ذلك الفصل أو معناه راجع تلك المقالة بســهولة فيجد ذلك الفصــل إمّا أن يجده كلام جالينوس أو معظمه أو يجــد ذلــك المعنى بلا نقص فيه ولا زيادة فــي كلام جالينوس في تلك المقالة وإن اختلفت العبارة فيرتفع الشكّ.

وليــس لأحد أن يعترضني في كوني أعــرف أنّ هذا الفصل ذكره جالينوس في المقالة الفلانية يكون جالينوس قد ذكر معنى ذلك الفصل أيضا في مقالة أخرى أو كرّره فــي عدّة مواضع لأنّي لو أحلتــه على أحد تلك المواضع للزم الاعتراض بعينه. وذكر المواضع كلّها فضل لا فائدة فيه أصلا بل تكثير كلام. لكنّي استحســنت عبارته عن ذلــك المعنى الكثير التكرار في كلامه في موضع من تلك المواضع فأثبتّه. فلا يلزمني أيضا اعتراض بأن يقال كيف وضعت فصلا في معنى كذا فلم تضع فصولا في المعنى الفلاني والمعنى الفلاني إذ غرض كلّ من ألّف فصولا كما ذكرت ليس هو الحصر. فإن قصــد قاصد لفصل من هذه الفصول واعترض وقال ما القصد في تقييد هذا الفصل

---

١ قوليهمــا] قولهمــا S | بقــراط] ابقراط LBP | معنى] om. LP || ٢ بنصّ] نصّ LBP || ٣ لــم] مــا S || ٤ مــن] من في G : فــي E || ٦ كلام] كتاب E || ٧ بيّن] يتبيّن SL : تبين EBP || ٨ أن يجــده] نــص L : نــص add. P | يجــده] نــص add. B | أو] أن add. E || ١٠ فيرتفع] ليرتفع E || ١٦ فصلا . . . تضع] om. E

concerning such and such an idea without adducing aphorisms concerning such and such another idea?" For no one who composes aphorisms has—as I have said—the intention to encompass [everything]. Therefore, if someone would consider one of these aphorisms and make an objection by saying: "What is the intention behind recording this aphorism but not that aphorism?" If you have recorded it so that it may be retained [in the memory], it is [an aphorism that is] very famous and well known among those practicing this art and does not need to be repeated. Similarly, about another aphorism one might say: "That aphorism you consider to be of peculiar interest is not of peculiar interest, in my opinion." And, similarly, one might say about yet another aphorism that I recorded because [I thought it to be] unknown: "There is no physician who does not know it." My answer to these objections would be that no person makes a selection for someone else, but he does so for himself in particular.

I have selected these aphorisms for myself only, so that I would have a ready record of them. Similarly, anyone who is like me or who is less knowledgeable than I am can benefit from them. I have not selected them for the benefit of someone who is at the same level as Galen or close to it. I have no doubt that many of these aphorisms are so [much more] clear[10] to others than to me, that they do not have to be learned by heart. Similarly, what I consider to be of peculiar interest may be not of peculiar interest for someone else, and what I consider to be mostly unknown may be well known to someone else. And [in] every [case] concerning which I think that I have solved a difficulty, either through the accurate account of [certain] ideas or through clarifying [certain] meanings,[11] there may be someone else for whom that difficulty does not arise in any respect because of his perfection in the art.

In these aphorisms I have included personal remarks, in which I have included only the [most] essential [additional information]. To these I refer in my own name. I have also included aphorisms from some of the later [physicians], which I attribute to the one who has presented them. I have divided these aphorisms into a number of treatises so that it will be easy to remember them or to show what one wants to show. I have made twenty-five treatises of them.

The first treatise contains aphorisms which concern the subject of the [medical] art, by which I mean the form of the organs of the human body [and] their functions and faculties. The second treatise contains aphorisms concerning the humors. The third treatise contains aphorisms

دون غيره إن كان قيّدته ليحفظ فهذا مشـــهور جدّا معلوم عند أهل هذه الصناعة لا يحتاج إلى تكرار . وكذلك يقول في فصل آخر هذا الذي ظننته غريبا ليس هو عندي بالغريب وكذلك يقول في فصل آخر قيّدته أنا لكونه ممّا يُجهل أنّه لا يجهل هذا طبيب . فجواب هذا الاعتراض أنّ الإنسان لا يختار لغيره وإنّما يختار لنفسه .

وهذه الفصول إنّما اخترتها لنفســي كالتذكرة وكذلك يستنفع بها كلّ من هو مثلي أو دوني في المعرفة . وما اخترتها ليســتنفع بها من هو في مرتبة جالينوس أو قريب منه . فلا شكّ عندي أنّ فصولا كثيرة من هذه الفصول هي عند غيري من البيان في حيّــز لا يحتاج إليها حفظ . وكذلك ما ظننته أنا غريبا يكون عند غيري غير غريب ومــا أظنّه أنا أنّه كثيرا ما يجهل يكون غيــري لا يجهله . وكلّ ما أرى أنا أنّي رفعت به إشــكالا إمّا في تحرير معان أو تبيين مدلولات يكون غيري لا يقع له ذلك الإشكال بوجعه لكماله في الصناعة .

وقد أتيت في هذه الفصول بأقاويل لي لخسّــتها فأذكرها باســمي وكذلك أتيت بفصول لبعض المتأخّرين أنســبها إلى قائلها . وقد قسّــمت هذه الفصول لعدّة مقالات ليسهل حفظها أو كشف ما يراد كشفه منها وجعلتها خمساً وعشرين مقالة .

المقالة الأولى تشــتمل على فصول تتعلّق بموضوع الصناعة أعني صورة أعضاء بدن الإنســان وأفعالها وقواها . المقالة الثانية تشـــتمل على فصول تتعلّق بالأخلاط .

---

١ إن كان] فهذه E : إن L | قيّدته] قيّده LB | عند أهل] لأهل B || ٢ تكرار] تذكار B || ٤ فجــواب] فيجــاب L : فيجب E || ٥ وكذلك] ولذلك SL || ٧ البيان] الثبات SLBP || ٨ إليهــا] لهــا ELP | أنــا] أنّــه B || ٩ أنــا] om. B | أنا] om. L || ١٠ إشــكالا] ما add. BP | مدلــولات] أســماء add. EL : أســمان add. B || ١١ لكمالــه] كماله (!)B || ١٢ أتيــت : أتــي L | بأقاويــل] بمعاني L | ١٢–١٣ بأقاويل . . . بفصــول] معاني E | لي لخسّتها . . . بفصول] om. L || ١٤ يراد] راد G || ١٥ صورة] om. SG

that concern the principles of the [medical] art and general rules. The fourth treatise contains aphorisms concerning the pulse and the prognostic signs to be derived from it. The fifth treatise contains aphorisms concerning the prognostic signs to be derived from the urine. The sixth treatise contains aphorisms concerning the other prognostic signs. The seventh treatise contains aphorisms concerning the causes [of diseases] which are often not known or which are discussed in a confused way. The eighth treatise contains aphorisms concerning the [correct] regimen for the healing of diseases in general. The ninth treatise contains aphorisms concerning specific diseases. The tenth treatise contains aphorisms concerning fevers. The eleventh treatise contains aphorisms concerning the periods and crisis of a disease. The twelfth treatise contains aphorisms concerning emptying [the body] by means of bloodletting. The thirteenth treatise contains aphorisms concerning evacuations by means of purgatives and enemas. The fourteenth treatise contains aphorisms concerning vomiting. The fifteenth treatise contains aphorisms concerning surgery. The sixteenth treatise contains aphorisms concerning women. The seventeenth treatise contains aphorisms concerning the regimen of health in general. The eighteenth treatise contains aphorisms concerning exercise. The nineteenth treatise contains aphorisms concerning bathing. The twentieth treatise contains aphorisms concerning foods and beverages[12] and their ingestion. The twenty-first treatise contains aphorisms concerning [natural] remedies. The twenty-second treatise contains aphorisms concerning [remedies with] special properties. The twenty-third treatise contains aphorisms on different diseases and symptoms whose names are

المقالة الثالثة تشتمل على فصول تتعلّق بأصول الصناعة وقوانين عامّة. المقالة الرابعة تشتمل على فصول تتعلّق بالنبض والاستدلال به. المقالة الخامسة تشتمل على فصول تتعلّق بالاستدلال بالبول. المقالة السادسة تشتمل على فصول تتعلّق بسائر الاستدلالات. المقالة السابعة تشتمل على فصول تتعلّق بإعطاء أسباب كثيرا ما تجهل أو يتشوّش القول فيها. المقالة الثامنة تشتمل على فصول تتعلّق بتدبير شفاء الأمراض على العموم. المقالة التاسعة تشتمل على فصول تتعلّق بأمراض مخصوصة. المقالة العاشرة تشتمل على فصول تتعلّق بالحمّيات. المقالة الحادية عشرة تشتمل على فصول تتعلّق بأوقات المرض وبحرانه. المقالة الثانية عشرة تشتمل على فصول تتعلّق بالاستفراغ بإخراج الدم. المقالة الثالثة عشرة تشتمل على فصول تتعلّق بالاستفراغ بأدوية مسهلة وحقن. المقالة الرابعة عشرة تشتمل على فصول تتعلّق بالقيء. المقالة الخامسة عشرة تشتمل على فصول تتعلّق بأعمال اليد. المقالة السادسة عشرة تشتمل على فصول تتعلّق بالنساء. المقالة السابعة عشرة تشتمل على فصول تتعلّق بتدبير الصحّة على العموم. المقالة الثامنة عشرة تشتمل على فصول تتعلّق بالرياضة. المقالة التاسعة عشرة تشتمل على فصول تتعلّق بالحمّام. المقالة العشرون تشتمل على فصول تتعلّق بالأغذية والمياه وتناولها. المقالة الحادية والعشرون تشتمل على فصول تتعلّق بالأدوية. المقالة الثانية والعشرون تشتمل على فصول تتعلّق بالخواصّ. المقالة الثالثة والعشرون تشتمل على فصول تتضمّن فروقا بين أمراض وأعراض مشهورة أسماؤها

---

٩ [١] بالاستفراغ] بالاستفراغات B | بإخراج] وبإخراج S : بخروج ELP | [٢] بالاستفراغ] بالاستفراغات B || ١١ بأعمال اليد] بالعمل باليد E || ١٣ الصحّة] الأصحّا E || ١٦ بالأدوية] بالأغذية (!)B || ١٧ وأعراض] .om. B

well known, and the elucidation of the meanings of those names which are known to the physicians, though sometimes not accurately. The twenty-fourth treatise contains curiosities related in the medical books, and unusual, rare occurrences. The twenty-fifth treatise contains doubts that occurred to me in different places due to Galen's words.

وتبيين معاني أســماء مشــهورة عند الأطبّاء قد يجهل معناها على التحرير. المقالة الرابعة والعشــرون تشــتمل على نوادر جرت وحكيت في كتب الطبّ وعلى أمور شــاذّة قليلة الوقوع. المقالة الخامســة والعشرون تشتمل على شكوك حدثت لي في مواضع من كلام جالينوس.

---

١ أســماء] om. SB | معناها] معانيها EL || ٢ نوادر] فصول L | وحكيت: om. B || ٣ لي] om. B || ٤ جالينوس] تمّ إحصاء المقالات بعون اللّه وتوفيقه امين add. B

The First Treatise

Containing aphorisms concerning the subject of the [medical] art, by which I mean the form of the organs of the human body [and] their functions and faculties

(1) The nerve which conveys to the muscle the faculty of sensation and movement from the brain and spinal cord is inserted into every muscle either at its head or between its beginning and middle [. . .], so that the middle is the head of that muscle. *De usu partium* 7.[1]

(2) The muscle called the diaphragm has its head in its center—namely, the sinewy place of the diaphragm to which the parts and ends of the nerves are attached[2] [. . .].[3] This is the line which encircles the diaphragm.[4] *De usu partium* 13.[5]

(3) Arteries and veins in the whole body are connected with[6] all the parts that [need][7] connection [with them]. They are near one another and sometimes so close together that the veins are in contact with the arteries. Thus, one always finds the veins directly upon the arteries, with the sole exception of the brain;[8] for the arteries ascend to it from below to facilitate the upward movement of the pneuma, while the veins descend

المقالة الأولى

تشتمل على فصول تتعلّق بموضوع الصناعة
أعني صورة أعضاء بدن الإنسان وأفعالها وقواها .

١ . العصب الذي يأتي العضل بقوة الحسّ والحركة من الدماغ ومن النخاع يتّصل بكلّ عضلة إمّا في أوّلها وإمّا في ما بين أوّلها ووسطها ويكون موضع الوسط هو رأس تلك العضلة . سابعة المنافع .

٢ . العضلة التي تسمّى الحجاب رأسها في وسطها وهو الموضع العصبي للحجاب الذي به تتّصل أقسام العصب وأطرافها هو الخطّ المحيط بدائرة الحجاب . ثالثة عشرة المنافع .

٣ . العروق الضوارب وغير الضوارب في جميع البدن تتّصل بالأعضاء التي ⟨تحتاج أن⟩ تتّصل بها . وهي متجاورة وربّما بلغ بها القرب أن يمسّ العرق الغير ضارب للضارب . وتجد العرق الغير ضارب أبدا موضوعا فوق العرق الضارب إلا الدماغ وحده فإنّ العروق الضوارب تصعد إليه من أسفل لسهولة حركة الروح للعلو والعروق

---

٥ ما] om. B | موضع] الموضع ELBP || ٧ للحجاب] من الحجاب SELBP ||
١٠ ⟨تحتاج أن⟩] Galen, *De usu part.*, fol. 157a | أن يمسّ] من B

to the brain from the crown of the head to facilitate the transport[9] of food to the brain. *De usu partium* 9.[10]

(4) To all the parts of the body come arteries and veins from the places that are nearest. But the testes and breasts are distinguished from all the parts of the body by the fact that the vessels that reach them do not come from nearby vessels, but from vessels that are far away, [in order] to prolong the [time that] the blood stays [in the vessels] so that the sperm and the milk will be completely cocted.[11] *De usu partium* 16.[12]

(5) Veins hidden from the eye reach the bones.[13] One does not find any muscle in the body that is devoid of veins and arteries. Nowhere is there an artery without a vein, but a few veins branch off without arteries; this happens close to the skin in the external parts of the body, in the hands, feet, and neck. *De usu partium* 16.[14]

(6) Branches of the arteries and small branches of nerves are intertwined with one another. Therefore, if the nerves are stretched,[15] the arteries share in the pain. *De pulsu* 10.[16]

(7) Someone who is not knowledgeable in anatomy supposes the round ligaments and tendons to be nerves. I would also have been unable to distinguish between them if I had not occupied myself with anatomical dissection. *De methodo medendi* 6.[17]

(8) No part of a nerve is attached to cartilage, ligaments, fat, or bones. The only exceptions among all the bodily parts are the teeth, for soft nerves are attached to their roots. Similarly, no nerves are attached to all glands which serve as a filling and foundation [for the division of vessels]. But glands needed for the necessary generation of fluids do have

الغير الضوارب تنحدر إلى الدماغ من أعلى الرأس ليسهل سيلان الغذاء إلى الدماغ. تاسعة المنافع.

٤ . الأعضــاء كلّها تأتيها العروق الضــوارب وغير الضوارب من أقرب المواضع منها . وقد خصّ الأنثيان والثديان دون جميع الأعضاء بأنّ ما يأتيها من العروق ليس يأتيهــا من العروق القريبة منها بل من البعيدة منها ليطول مكث الدم هناك حتى ينضج المني واللبن غاية النضج . سادسة عشرة المنافع .

٥ . يأتي العظام عروق غير ضوارب تخفى عن البصر ولا تجد في البدن شــيئًا من العضل يخلو عن عرق غير ضارب وضارب . ولا يوجد عرق ضارب في موضع من المواضع إلا ومعه عرق غير ضارب ، وأمّا العروق غير الضوارب فإنّ يســيرا منها ينقسم ولا يوجد معه عرق ضارب ، وذلك قريب من الجلد في ظاهر البدن في اليدين وفي الرجلين وفي الرقبة. سادسة عشرة المنافع .

٦ . شــعب العروق الضوارب وشــعب العصب الجزئية يخالط بعضها بعضا . فلذلك متى تمدّد جنس العصب شاركته العروق الضوارب في الألم. عاشرة النبض .

٧ . الرباطات المدوّرة والأوتار يظنّ من لا بصر له بالتشريح أنّ ذلك عصب . ولا نحن كنّا أيضا نعرف واحدا منها لولا علاج التشريح . سادسة الحيلة .

٨ . العصب لا يتّصل شــيء منه بغضروف ولا برباط ولا بشــحم ولا بعظم إلا بالأسنان وحدها من جميع العظام فإنّها يتّصل بأصولها عصب ليّن . وكذلك لا يتّصل العصب بشــيء من الغدد الذي يقوم مقام الحشــو والدعامة . أمّا الغدد المحتاج إليها

---

٧ العظام] العضل G | البصر] النظر LP : حسّ E || ٨ عن] من EL || ١٣ جنس] جسم ELB[1] || ١٤ المــدوّرة] om. L | ١٤–١٥ المــدوّرة . . . الحيلــة] om. E | ١٤ بصر] نظر B || ١٨ الغدد] الجلد B

a few nerves attached to them in a few rare cases, just as they also have arteries and veins. *De usu partium* 16.[18]

(9) Tendons are softer than ligaments but harder than nerves. The volume of[19] the substance of a tendon is [equal] to that of a ligament[20] and nerve together. In many places within muscles, one finds [the size of] a ligament to be ten times that of a nerve that is attached to that muscle at its head. Every nerve is sensitive, but no ligament has sensation. Every tendon has less sensation than a nerve because it is in part a ligament.[21] *De motu musculorum* 1.[22]

(10) The body has three structures[23] which are similar[24] in bodily form. One of these is the nerve, another is the ligament, and a third is the tendon. A tendon is one of the two ends of a muscle and resembles a nerve. It is the product of nerve and ligament. Every nerve is exactly round, but not all the tendons are like that; some of them are round and others are somewhat flat. Most[25] of them become so wide that they resemble a membrane. *De placitis Hippocratis et Platonis* 1.9.[26]

(11) All membranes are extremely thin and soft, but a ligament is mostly hard and thick. Some ligaments are in between the nature of nerves and cartilage. But no membrane or nerve or tendon can approach anywhere [near] to the hardness of a ligament; similarly, the hardest nerve cannot achieve the hardness of a tendon. *Ibidem.*[27]

لتوليد الرطوبة المحتاج إليها فقد يتّصل بها في الندرة يسير عصب كما يوجد فيها أيضا عروق ضوارب وغير ضوارب. سادسة عشرة المنافع.

٩. الوتر ألين من الرباط وأصلب من العصب. ومقدار عظم جرم الوتر هو المقدار الذي يكون من الرباط والعصب مجموعين. وفي مواضع كثيرة من العضل تجد الوتر عشرة أمثال العصبة التي اتّصلت بتلك العضلة من رأسها. وكلّ عصب حسّاس وكلّ رباط غير حسّاس. وكلّ وتر فحسّه دون حسّ العصب بحسب ما خالطه من الرباط. في الأول من حركات العضل.

١٠. في الجسم ثلاث آلات متقاربة الحال في صور أجرامها. أحدها عصب والآخر رباط والثالث وتر. والوتر هو أحد طرفي العضلة وهو عصباني. وتولّده يكون من العصب والرباطات. وكلّ العصب مستدير محكم الاستدارة وليس الأوتار كلّها كذلك بل منها مدوّر ومنها منبسط قليلا. أمّا الرباطات فأكثر ما تعترض حتى تصير شبيهة بالغشاء. في الأولى من آراء ابقراط وافلاطون.

١١. الأغشية كلّها في غاية الرقّة واللين وأمّا الرباط فهو في أكثر الحالات صلب غليظ. وبعض الرباطات فيما بين طبيعة العصب والغضروف. وليس ثمّ لا غشاء ولا عصبة ولا وتر يصير في موضع من المواضع في صلابة الرباط، وكذلك أصلب ما يكون من العصب لا ينتهي إلى صلابة الوتر. في تلك المقالة.

١–٧ الوتر . . . خالطه] om. P || ٨ الجسم] البدن ELBP || ١٠ والرباطات] والرباط L || ١١ فأكثر ما] فأكثرها B | تعترض] تعرض ELP : يعرض B || ١٤ ثمّ] لا add. EL

(12) These three structures—namely, nerve, tendon, and ligament—are all white, solid, and bloodless. If you dissect them, they separate into lengthwise[28] fibers, except for the very hard ligaments, for [these] cannot be taken apart into fibers. *De placitis Hippocratis et Platonis* 1.[29]

(13) A muscle is an instrument for motion only and not for sensation, because every voluntary motion occurs exclusively through a muscle. Everything that is not a muscle has sensation, because everything to which a nerve is attached has sensation, even though it has no voluntary motion. *Ibidem.*[30]

(14) The ligaments[31] with which muscles are attached to bones give rise to membranes that envelop the muscles and from which strands[32] spread into the flesh of the muscles. *Ibidem.*[33]

(15) Every tendon is attached to a bone for the most part, but not every muscle ends in a tendon, for none of the muscles which move the tongue and the lips and the eyes has a tendon, since [these muscles] do not move a bone. Most of the parts of the face move voluntarily, while the bones are motionless and do not need tendons. *Ibidem.*[34]

(16) If someone rapidly suffers from an obstruction[35] in the liver, it happens because the ends of the vessels in which the food arises from the concave side of the liver to the convex side are narrow. *De alimentorum facultatibus* 3.[36]

(17) The constitutions of bodies that are extremely susceptible to illness are, in particular, those composed of parts with an opposite temperament. An example of this is [the case where] the stomach is extremely hot and the brain is cold. Similarly, the lungs and entire chest are often cold while the stomach is hot, and frequently the opposite is the case. Many times, the other parts are cold and the liver is extremely hot. One should suspect the very same thing to be true for the other parts [of the body]. *De alimentorum facultatibus* 3.[37]

١٢ . هــذه الثلاث الآلات وهي العصبة والوتر والرباط كلّها بيض مصمتة عادمة الــدم . إذا حللتها انحلت إلى ليف ذاهب في الطول خلا ما كان من الرباطات صلبا جدّا فإنّه لا يمكن أن ينحل فيصير ليفا . الأولى من آراء ابقراط وافلاطون .

١٣ . العضلــة هي آلة للحركة فقط وليس هي آلة للحسّ لأنّ كلّ حركة إرادية لا تكــون إلا بعضلة . وقد يحسّ ما ليس هو عضلة لأنّ كلّ ما يتّصل به العصب يحسّ وإن لم يكن له حركة إرادية . في تلك المقالة .

١٤ . الرباطات التي يرتبط بها العضل بالعظام هي تولد الأغشــية التي تغشــى العضل وينبعث شعب منها إلى داخل في لحم العضل . في تلك المقالة .

١٥ . كلّ وتر فإنّه يتّصل بعظم في أكثر الأمر وليس كلّ عضلة ينتهي إلى وتر . لأنّ العضل المحرّك للسان والمحرّك للشفتين والعينين لا يوجد لواحدة منها وتر لأنّها لا تحرّك عظما . وأكثر أعضاء الوجه تتحرّك بإرادة والعظام ساكنة فلا تحتاج لأوتار . في تلك المقالة .

١٦ . والذي يســرع الســدد إلى كبده هو من كانت أطراف العروق التي يصعد الغذاء فيها من الجانب المقعّر من الكبد إلى الجانب المحدّب ضيّقة . ثالثة الأغذية .

١٧ . هيئات الأبدان التي هي مســتقامة غاية الســقم إنّما هي مركّبة من أعضاء متضــادّة المزاج . وذلك بأن تكون المعدة في المثــل حارّة غاية الحرارة والدماغ باردا . وكذلك كثيرا ما يكون الرئة وجملة الصدر باردين والمعدة حارّة وكثيرا ما يكون الأمر على خلاف ذلك . وكثيرا ما تكون سائر الأعضاء باردة وتكون الكبد أسخن فتوهّم هذا بعينه في سائر الأعضاء . ثالثة الأغذية .

---

٨ وينبعث شعب] وتبعث شعبا ELBP || ١١ والعظام] والعظم L || ١٦ على خلاف ذلك] بالخلاف EL

(18) At every place in the body where a nerve or tendon has to pass through the large protuberance of a bone, one of these three things necessarily occurs: either a groove is made into the bone [to receive it], or [the bone] is pierced through, or the nerve or tendon encircles the bone—but it never extends bare over the convexity of the bone. All the nerves, tendons, and veins which lie in bony grooves are covered and protected by strong membranes. *De usu partium* 2.[38]

(19) Within arteries and veins are two parts:[39] blood and pneuma, [which remain] separate except that a little thin, vaporous blood flows in the arteries, while a little mistlike pneuma flows in the veins.[40] Arteries in the whole body communicate with veins and exchange blood and pneuma through certain invisible narrow passages. *De usu partium* 6.[41]

(20) In his treatise *On the Usefulness of the Pulse,* [Galen] said: "The arteries return a small amount to the heart during their contraction."[42] The thinnest and lightest [substance] in the body is pneuma, followed in second place by vapor, followed in third place by thin, completely[43] cocted blood. *De naturalibus facultatibus* [3].[44]

(21) Organs that are [generally] considered unpaired in the body are in reality paired, such as the brain, the tongue, the jawbone, the lung, the chest,[45] the womb, and their like; for the number of parts in the right side of each of these organs is equal to that in the left side. These parts are likewise equal in their dimensions, thickness, thinness, and external form, and their whole nature never changes. Similarly, the category of arteries, veins, and nerves that come to one side of these organs is similar to that [which come to] the other side. *De providentia creatoris.*[46]

١٨ . كلّ موضع من البدن يحتاج أن يمرّ عصبة أو وتر بطرف عظم كبير فلا بدّ من أحد ثلاث خصال : إمّا أن يحزّ في العظم أو يثقب أو يلتفّ عليه العصبة أو الوتر ولا يمرّ على حدبة العظم وهو مكشوف أصلا . وجميع الأعصاب والأوتار والعروق الموضوعة في المواضع المحزوزة من العظام مغطاة موقاة بأغشية قوية . ثانية المنافع .

١٩ . في العروق الضوارب وغير الضوارب الدم والروح جزءان إلا أنّ ما في العروق الضوارب من الدم قليل لطيف قريب من طبيعة البخار والذي في العروق الغير ضوارب من الروح يسير ضبابي . والعروق الضوارب في جميع البدن نافذة إلى العروق الغير ضوارب يأخذ بعضها من بعض دما وروحا من منافذ خفية عن البصر ضيّقة . في سادسة المنافع .

٢٠ . وقال في مقالته في منفعة النبض إنّ العروق الضوارب تردّ إلى القلب شيئا يسيرا عند انقباضها . ألطف ما في البدن وأخفّه الروح ثمّ الثاني بعده البخار ثمّ الثالث بعدها الدم المحكم النضج اللطيف . ثالثة القوى .

٢١ . الأعضاء التي تظنّ بها أنّها في البدن مفردة هي بالحقيقة زوج مثل الدماغ واللسان واللحي والرئة والصدر والرحم وغيرها ، ممّا أشبهها . فإنّ ما في الجانب الأيمن من كلّ واحد منها فيه عدد من الأجزاء مساو لما في الجانب الأيسر منها ، وكذلك تلك الأجزاء متساوية في مقاديرها وثخنها ورقّتها ولونها وجميع طبعها لا تختلف أصلا . وكذلك جنس العروق الضوارب وغير الضوارب والعصب التي تأتي كلّ جانب منها مثل التي تأتي الجانب الآخر . في مقالته في عناية الخالق .

---

١ يحتاج] إلى add. ELBP || ٤ المواضع] من المواضع add. L | المحروزة] المحزوزة L || ٥ جزئان] موجودان Galen, *De usu part.* || ٧.١١–١٢.١٧ الروح . . . إذا أردت إبقاء العضو ممدودا] om. B || ١٤ فإنّ . . . منها] فإن كان في الجانب الأيمن هو بعينه في الجانب الأيسر EL || ١٧ جنس] جسم EL

(22) Although the tongue seems from the outside to be a single organ, in reality it is double, since each half of it lengthwise has its own specific arteries, veins, and nerves attached to it. Similarly, the muscles of one half are different from those of the other half. No muscle, vein, artery, or nerve passes in it from the right side to the left side or from the left side to the right side. *De usu partium* 11.[47]

(23) When a small nerve must be conducted over a long distance or when it is responsible for the vigorous movement of a muscle, that small nerve is strengthened and supported by a substance that is thicker than the substance of the nerve, although similar to it.[48] If you look at it, you might think[49] that it has become rounded and that it is attached to the nerve and intertwined with it. But it is not[50] attached to the nerve, nor joined to it. When the nerve thickens with that substance, you will see that the nerve extending from it has a large diameter. *De usu partium* 16.[51]

(24) There are altogether four [different] kinds of movements of a muscle, namely [these]: it is either contracted, or [it is] extended, or [it is] twisted,[52] or it remains stretched and tense. The first and the fourth kinds [of movement] are characteristic functions of all muscles. *De motu musculorum* 1.[53]

(25) Says Moses: A summary of his words about these four movements is [thus]: When one's will sends the psychical faculty through a nerve to the muscle with which it wants to flex a specific limb, that muscle contracts toward its origin, so that that limb is flexed. Similarly, when one wants that limb to remain stretched and raised, the will stretches that muscle, together with its antagonistic muscle,[54] so that they both

٢٢ . اللسان وإن كان يرى واحدا في الظاهر فإنّه بالحقيقة اثنان لأنّ كلّ نصف منه على طوله تتّصل به وحده عروق ضوارب وغير ضوارب وعصب تخصّه. وكذلك عضل هذا الشقّ منه غير عضل الشقّ الآخر. ولا تنفذ فيه عضلة ولا عرق غير ضارب ولا ضارب ولا عصبة من الجانب الأيمن إلى الأيسر ولا من الأيسر إلى الأيمن. حادية عشرة المنافع.

٢٣ . متى احتيج أن يسلك بعصبة صغيرة مسافة بعيدة أو توكّل بتحريك عضلة قوية الحركة قويت تلك العصبة الصغيرة وعضدت بجرم أغلظ من جرم العصب وهو شبيه بجوهر العصب. وأنت إذا رأيته تظنّه عصبة مدوّرة وتظنّه ملتزقا بتلك العصبة ملتفّا معها. وليس هو ملتزق مع العصبة ولا متّصل بها . فإذا غلظت العصبة بذلك الجوهر رأيت العصبة التي تمتدّ بعدها عظيمة الاستدارة. سادسة عشرة المنافع.

٢٤ . جميع أصناف حركات العضل أربعة وذلك أنّه إمّا أن ينقبض وإمّا أن ينبسط وإمّا أن ينفتل وإمّا أن يبقى ممدودا موتّرا . فالصنف الأوّل والرابع هو فعل خاصّ بجميع العضل. في أولى من كتاب حركات العضل.

٢٥ . قال موسى الذي تلخّص من قوله في هذه الأربع حركات هو أنّ الإرادة إذا أرسلت القوة النفسانية في العصب نحو عضلة من العضل تريد أن تثني بها ذلك العضو تقلّصت تلك العضلة نحو مبدئها فانثنى ذلك العضو. وكذلك إذا أرادت إبقاء العضو ممدودا مشالا مددت الإرادة تلك العضلة مع العضلة المقابلة لها وتوتّرا جميعا .

---

١ بالحقيقة] في الحقيقة SL || ٣ منه غير عضل الشقّ] om. L || ٧ وهو] في سائر حالاته بعد الغلظ add. Galen, *De usu part.* || ٨ مدوّرة] وفي أوّل وقوع البصر عليه وتخيله add. Galen, *De usu part.* || ٩ وليس] حتى إذا شرحته علمت علما يقينا أنّه ليس add. Galen, *De usu part.* || ١١ ينفتل] يفتل S : يثقل P || ١٦ وكذلك] ولذلك GB | أرادت] أردت SG

become tense. And when one's will ceases its activity altogether and no longer sends any force to the muscle, the muscle becomes[55] like the other inert things, and because of its natural weight, it falls downward, [along] with that bone to which it is connected, like a lifeless limb. This movement attributed to the muscle is not caused by the activity of the muscle and is therefore not counted among the voluntary movements. The movement of extension is a voluntary and deliberate movement of the muscle; for when one's will wants to stretch a flexed limb, it stops the psychical faculty in the flexed, contracted muscle and sends it to the antagonistic muscle. The result is that the antagonistic muscle is contracted and the first muscle, which had [initially] flexed the limb, is stretched, since the power which prevented it from doing so is no longer there. If we want to stretch it as far as possible, we must use the psychical faculty to achieve this.

(26) Any muscle stretches a limb only when that limb is flexed. Similarly, any muscle flexes a limb only when it is stretched. A limb is flexed by the internal muscle and stretched by the external muscle. Therefore, if either one of them is severed, both movements are abolished altogether—that is to say, the limb will not be flexed[56] or stretched endlessly [anymore] but will remain in one position, according to the healthy muscle which effects that position. *De motu musculorum* 1.[57]

(27) When we sleep, the positions of our limbs are always between the extreme position and intermediate position; the activity of the muscles is not abolished at that time. When someone is asleep while he is drunk or very tired or weak, he causes all the limbs of his body to be extremely relaxed; his muscles are in the intermediate position and are completely at rest during sleep. *De motu musculorum* 2.[58]

وإن عطّلت الإرادة فعلها بالجملة ولم ترسل للعضل قوة أصلا بقيت العضل شبه سائر الجمادات فتهوى بثقلها الطبيعي مع ذلك العظم الذي هي منوّطة به إلى الأسفل كالعضو الميّت. وهذه الحركة تنسب للعضل ليس من أجل أنّها من فعل العضل ولذلك لا تعدّ من الحركات الإرادية. فأمّا حركة الانبساط فهي إرادية وهي حركة للعضلة بالغرض وذلك أنّ الإرادة إذا أرادت أن تبسط العضو المثني عطّلت القوة النفسانية من العضلة التي اثنت متقلّصة وأرسلت تلك القوة للعضلة المقابلة لها. فانقبضت تلك المقابلة فتنبسط الأولى التي كانت أثنت العضو إذ لم تبق فيها قوة ممانعة. وإذا أردنا التبسّط في الغاية استعملت القوة النفسانية بسط العضلة في الغاية.

٢٦. كلّ عضلة تبسط عضوا ما إنّما تبسطه إذا كان منثنيا. وكذلك كلّ عضلة تثنيه إنّما تثنيه إذا كان منبسطا. والعضو ينثني بالعضل الداخل وينبسط بالخارج. فلذلك إن قطعت أحدهما تعطّلت الحركتان جميعا أعني أنّه لا يبقى ينقبض وينبسط بل يبقى على وضع واحد بحسب العضلة السالمة التي تفعل ذلك الوضع. في تلك المقالة.

٢٧. الأشكال التي بين الشكل الذي في الغاية وبين الشكل الأوسط هي أبدا أشكال أعضائنا إذا كنّا تيّاما وليس فعل العضل فيها حينئذ متعطّل. أمّا من نيام وبه سكر أو تعب شديد أو ضعف فإنّه يرخى جميع أعضاء بدنه غاية الإرخاء وتصير العضل في الأوسط فتكون ساكنة سكونا تامّا عند النوم. في الثانية من حركات العضل.

---

١ العضل] العضلة EL || ٣ ولذلك] وكذلك G || ٤ فأمّا . . . فهي إرادية] .om B | إرادية وهي] om. EL | للعضلة] العضلة LB || ٥ بالغرض conj. Bos] بالعرض BEGLPS | المثني] المنثني B | عطّلت] عملت (!)B || ٨ التبسّط] البسط SEBP || ٩ إنّما] أن add. G || ١٠ إنّما تثنيه] om. EL || ١٢ الوضع] الفعل L : به E || ١٣ بين] من G | وبين] ومن G || ١٤ كنّا تيّاما] كانت نائمة EL | نيام] نام EL

(28) The muscles of the anus, the urinary bladder, and the diaphragm are all round. Those around the urinary bladder and around the anus were not created for expelling superfluities, as [some] people think, but for retaining them; for they retain the superfluities and prevent them from streaming when it is not the [proper] time. But when one's will lets them go and releases them so that they are no [longer] retained and restrained, then the superfluities are expelled by the natural expulsive faculties, which receive help from the action of the abdominal muscles and from the stretching of the diaphragm. *De motu musculorum* 2.[59]

(29) When the diaphragm becomes tense, as all muscles do—that is to say, when it contracts and draws together—the inhalation of air becomes easy. When it extends from this contraction, which occurs when the abdominal muscles contract alone or when the muscles between the ribs contract alone, exhalation becomes easy. *De motu musculorum* 2.[60]

(30) The diaphragm alone effects inhalation and exhalation easily. Difficult exhalation and inhalation is effected by the muscles between the ribs and the muscles that reach the chest from[61] the shoulders and neck. *De motu musculorum* 2.[62]

(31) Every individual muscle carries the bone to which it is attached as if it were carrying a stone; and, as long as it is strong, it is capable of doing so. For the most part, then, it does not feel its burden—not even a little bit. But, when [a muscle] is weak, it feels its burden and it is hard for [the muscle] to carry it. It is as if [the muscle] would like to push it away and to transfer it from one position to another.[63] This is the reason why ill people change the position of their limbs every moment and cannot bear one [consistent] position. *De motu musculorum* 1.[64]

٢٨ . العضلــة التي في المقعدة والتي في المثانة والتي في الحجاب كلّ واحدة من هذه مدوّرة . وأمّا التي حول المثانة وحول المقعدة فلم تخلق لدفع الفضول كما ظنّ قوم بل خلقت لحبســها وهي حابسة مانعة لسيلان الفضول في غير وقتها . وإذا أطلقتها الإرادة وتخلّــت عن الحبــس والمنع دفعت حينئذ الفضول بالقــوى الدافعة الطبيعية ويعينه فعل العضل الذي على البطن وتوتّر الحجاب . في تلك المقالة .

٢٩ . إذا توتّر الحجاب التوتّرالذي هو فعل جميع العضل أعني تقلّصه واجتماعه دخل النفس رسيلا . وإذا انبسط من ذلك التقلّص وذلك عند ما يتقلّص عضل البطن وحدها أو عند ما يتقلّص العضل الذي بين الأضلاع وحده خرج النفس رسيلا . في تلك المقالة .

٣٠ . الحجاب وحده يفعل دخول النفس وخروجه رســلا . وأمّا خروج النفس بشــدّة ودخول النفس بشدّة فإنّ العضل الذي في ما بين الأضلاع والعضل الذي يأتي الصدر بين الكتفين والرقبة يفعلهما . في تلك المقالة .

٣١ . كلّ واحدة من العضل تحمل العظم الملتحم بها كأنّها تحمل حجرا فما دامت قوية فإنّها لا تعيا به . وأكثر ذلك لا تحسّ بثقله ولا الحسّ اليسير . فإذا ضعفت فإنّها تحسّ حينئذ بثقله فيشــتدّ عليها حمله . وكأنّها تحبّ دفعه عنها فتتوّق إلى نقله من شــكل إلى شــكل . وهذه هي العلّة في كون المرضى يغيّرون شكل أعضائهم في كلّ قليل ولا يحتملون الصبر على شكل واحد . في الأولى من كتاب حركات العضل .

---

٤ وتخلّت] وكلت EL || ٧ رسـيلا] رسـلا ELP || ٨ النفس] التنفس EL | رسـيلا] رسـلا ELP || ١٠–١٢ الحجـاب . . . فـي تلك المقالـة] om. E | ١٠ النفـس] التنفس L | وخروجـه . . . خروج النفس] om. B | رسـلا] رسـيلا S | النفـس] التنفس L || ١١ النفس] التنفس L | بين] من LBP

(32) All the activities of the muscles become weak during sleep. Only the activity of the muscles that move the chest stays the same. *De locis affectis* 5.[65]

(33) Do not be surprised that most people, when asleep, perform most voluntary activities, such as speaking, screaming, walking, and turning from side to side; for [even] those who are awake perform [their] activities in a state of absentmindedness, such that one may be on one's way with the intention of reaching a certain place while one is absentminded and does not know where one is going until the journey is completed. *De motu musculorum* 2.[66]

(34) Says Moses: These voluntary activities that one who is asleep and one who is absentminded perform have been extensively verified by Galen in this treatise by his description of his observations, but he [verifies the phenomenon] without giving a reason for it. Neither did he resolve the doubt[67]—although it calls for a solution—raised by the following question: How can the will of someone who is asleep or absentminded be nullified and yet [direct] him to carry out voluntary movements? Galen [himself] confirmed his perplexity and doubt about these movements by saying: "Although we do not know the reasons for this, we cannot deny what we see with our own eyes." But I will give the reason for this in a summary, and it should be clear after the following introductory remarks.

(35) First introductory remark: Voluntary movements sometimes follow from thought and reflection, as in our movement to observe a certain star. At other times they follow from one's imagination, as, for instance, in the erection of someone's penis when he imagines a certain person.[68] At yet other times they follow from nature—in effect, a sensation—as, for instance, in the contraction of someone's leg when a flea bites him.

(36) Second introductory remark: All the voluntary movements of the other, nonrational animals follow from imagination or sensation.

٣٢ . أفعـال العضل كلّها في وقت النوم تفتر . وفعل العضل المحرّك للصدر وحده يكون باقيا على حاله . خامسة التعرّف .

٣٣ . لا تعجب من كون أكثر النيام يفعلون أكثر الأفعال الإرادية كالكلام والصياح والمشي والتقلب من جانب إلى جانب . فإنّ النبهان يفعل أفعالا وهو ساه عنها حتى أنّه يمشي في طريق يقصد موضعا ويمشي وهو ساه ولا يعلم حيث يمشي حتى يقطع الطريق كلّها . في الثانية من كتاب حركات العضل .

٣٤ . قال موسـى : هـذه الأفعال الإرادية التي يفعلها النائم والسـاهي قد طوّل جالينوس في تصحيح ذلك في هذه المقالة بإخباره بما شـاهد ولم يعط السـبب في ذلك . ولا حلّ الشّـك الذي يـروم حلّه وهو قولنا : كيف بطلـت الإرادة من النائم والسـاهي وهو يتحرّك الحركات الإرادية؟ وقد أقرّ جالينوس بالحيرة والشكّ في هذه الحركات وقال : وإن كنّا لا نعلم أسباب ذلك فلا نكذّب بما نشاهد . وأعطي السبب في ذلك بإيجاز يتبيّن بعد التنبيه على هذه المقدّمات .

٣٥ . مقدّمـة أولى : الحـركات الإرادية قد تكون تابعة لفكـرة وروية كحركتنا لرصد كوكب من الكواكب . وقد تكون تابعة لخيال ما كإنعاظ الإنسـان عند تخيّله شـخص ما . وقد تكون تابعة لطبيعة أعني الإحسـاس كقبض الإنسـان رجلة إذا قرصه برغوث .

٣٦ . مقدّمة ثانية : جميع حركات سـائر الحيـوان غير الناطق الإرادية إنّما هي تابعة لخيال أو من أجل الإحساس .

---

٣ أكثر] om. SGB ‖ ٨ شـاهد] يشـاهد LBP ‖ ٩ ولا حلّ] لأجل E ‖ ١٤ كإنعاظ] كإنعاص G ‖ ١٨ أو] om. B

(37) Third introductory remark: You know that the imaginative faculty is fully and completely active during sleep, as is the imaginative form[69] in the imagination of someone who is absentminded, even if he thinks of something else.

(38) Fourth introductory remark: It is well known that sensation is not nullified in living creatures when they are asleep, as Galen explained in this treatise.[70] However, it is diminished and is similar to the strength of someone who is resting and relaxing after great exertion and lassitude.

After these introductory remarks, it may be clear to you that all those activities which Galen mentioned [on the part] of those who are asleep result either from imagination only or from the nature of the sensation; for someone who is asleep will awaken if a light is brought close to his eyes, or he hears a loud noise, or he is pricked by a needle, or his body is overcome by strong heat or severe cold, or he is hungry or thirsty. Similarly, if he feels pain in one side [of his body], he turns to another side. All these are movements resulting from the nature [of the sensation]. It is not difficult for you [to understand] that a drunk person or someone who suffered from a stroke does not notice any of these, because they are not healthy, but ill. The activities resulting from sound thinking are totally nullified in the case of someone who is asleep. The walking of someone who is asleep or who is absentminded results from the imaginative form that initially occurred to the sleeper when he was awake and to the absentminded one when he was attentive.[71]

(39) We remember of our own accord the things we do and the words we say intentionally when we are healthy or when we are reminded of them [by others]. But drunken people and those with a very confused mind do not remember—once they have recovered—anything of the things they have done, even if one tries to remind them of them. *De motu musculorum* 2.[72]

٣٧ . مقدّمــة ثالثة : قد علمــت أنّ القوة الخيالية تفعل فعلها على الكمال والتمام في حــال النوم وكذلك الصورة الخيالية التي في خيال الســاهي وإن كان مفكرا في شيء آخر .

٣٨ . مقدّمــة رابعة : معلــوم أنّ الحسّ في الحيوان في حــال نومه لم يبطل كما بيّن جالينوس في هذه المقالة . لكنّه نقص وهو شــبه قوة من اســتراح من تعب شديد واسترخاء .

وبعــد هذه المقدّمات يتبيّن لــك أنّ كلّ ما ذكره جالينوس من أفعال النيام هو تابع إمّا لمجرّد الخيال أو لطبيعة الحاسّــة . لأنّ النائم إذا قرب الضوء من عينيه أو ســمع صوتا عظيما أو نخس بإبرة أو استولى على جسمه حرّ شديد أو برد شديد أو جاع أو عطــش انتبه . وكذلك إذا تألّم جانب انقلــب لجانب آخر . وهكذا كلّها حركات تابعة لطبيعة . ولا يعســر عليك كون الســكران أو المسكوت لا ينتبه لشيء من هذه لأنّ أولائــك مرضى لا أصحّاء . والتي تتعطّل من النائــم بالكلّية هي الأفعال التابعة لفكرة صحيحة . ومشــي النائم أو الساهي عند مشيه إنّما ذلك تابع للصورة الخيالية الحاصلــة أوّلا في حال اليقظة من الذي هو الآن نائم أو في حال القصد من الذي هو الآن ساه .

٣٩ . الأفعــال والأقاويل التي نفعلها بقصد وفي حال الســلامة نحن نذكرها من أنفسنا وإذا ذُكّرنا بها . وأمّا أفعال السكارى والمختلطي العقل اختلاطا عظيما فإنّهم لا يذكرون شيئًا منها إذا برؤوا ولو ذكّرناهم بها . في الثانية من كتاب حركات العضل .

---

٥ نقص] يقص B || ١١ ينتبه] ينتبهان EL || ١٨ بها] om. L

(40) Says Moses: The reason for this is that the retentive faculty retains [only] those things deposited in it intentionally and voluntarily by the healthy cogitative faculty.[73] You can find a confirmation for this in the fact that those things that we strongly intend to remember are better fixed in our retentive faculty than those we [do] not so strongly intend to remember.

Those who keep something in their hands while they are asleep provide clear proof that the movement of tension remains in their muscles, for their fingers continue to be clasped around a small object. [The fact] that healthy people keep their jaws closed during their sleep is also clear proof for the movement of tension [during their sleep]. Similarly, the muscle surrounding the place where the superfluities leave the body performs its function with great intensity in the case of those who are asleep. *De motu musculorum* 2.[74]

(41) The brain has a constant movement of contraction and expansion, just like the pulse in the measured movement of the arteries and the heart. This is clear in the case of small children and in the case of someone whose cranial bone is exposed.[75] If a living creature cries out loudly, the entire brain swells and expands. I suppose that the reason for this is that, at the time of the loud cry, superfluous heat increases and [superfluous] matters are compressed and tend upward. When the brain expands, air is attracted through the nostrils; and when it contracts, the vaporous superfluity and other superfluities that it contains are compressed and expelled from it. But the heat [of the brain] always remains well preserved there. *De instrumento odoratus.*[76]

(42) The thin brain membrane[77] adheres to the brain, whereas the thick, hard membrane[78] is separated from the thin membrane.[79] The only connections between them are the emerging vessels. The hard membrane is perforated by straight, solid holes, just like a sieve. These holes are constantly cleansed by the two aspects of respiration: inhalation and

٤٠ . قال موسى : السبب في ذلك أنّ القوة الحافظة إنّما تحفظ ما يودع فيها بقصد وبإرادة من القوة المفكّرة السالمة . وممّا يؤكد عندك كون الأشياء التي نعني بحفظها عناية شديدة أثبت في قوّتنا الحافظة من الأشياء التي تكون عنايتنا بحفظها أقلّ .

فصل . الذين يحفظون في أيديهم شيئا وهم نيام يدلّون دلالة بيّنة أنّ حركة التوتّر باقية في عضلهم وقد تبقى أصابعهم مضمومة على جسم صغير . وانضمام اللحيين أيضا في حال نوم الأصحّاء دليل واضح على فعل التوتّر في حال النوم . وكذلك العضل المطوّق بمخرج الفضول يفعل فعله بقوة شديدة في النيام . في الثانية من كتاب حركات العضل .

٤١ . الدماغ له دائما حركة انقباض وانبساط يجري مجرى النبض في وزن حركة العروق الضوارب والقلب . وذلك بيّن في الصبيان الصغار وفي من انكشف عظم من رأسه . وإذا صاح الحيوان ينتفخ الدماغ كلّه ويزيد . وأحسب أنّ السبب في ذلك أنّ عند الصياح الشديد ينشؤ فضل حرارته وأيضا أنّ الموادّ تتعصّر فتميل إلى فوق . وبانبساط الدماغ يجذب الهواء من المنخرين وبانقباضه يعصر على ما فيه من فضل دخاني وغيره من الفضلات فيخرجها عنه . وتبقى حرارته أبدا محروسة سالمة . في مقالته في آلة الشمّ .

٤٢ . غشاء الدماغ الرقيق لاصق بالدماغ والغشاء الثخين الصلب مباين للغشاء الرقيق . وليس بينه وبينه اتّصال إلا ما ينفذ فيه من العروق . والغشاء الصلب مثقّب ثقبا صلبة مستقيمة بمنزلة المصفاة . وتلك الثقب تنقّى بجزئي التنفّس كلّيهما تنقية

---

٧ العضــل] الفضــل (!)B || ١١ ينتفــخ] ينفتح (!)B || ١٢ فضــل حرارته] فعل الحرارة B || ١٧ بينه وبينه] بينهما E || ١٨ تنقّى] om. L | بجزئي] مجري SG : بجري LB : بجرو (?)E

exhalation. The bone which protects the brain and is close to the face and palate is hollow; the anatomists call it the "sieve."[80] Its openings are not straight, like those of a sieve, but have an irregular structure, as in a sponge, so that the air, when it is extremely cold and then inhaled, will not enter the ventricles of the brain straightway. *De usu partium* 8.[81]

(43) Between the bone of the upper palate and the hard brain membrane is a network woven from arteries.[82] This network lies underneath the entire brain, except for a small part thereof. It consists of many layers—as if you were to imagine many fishermen's nets spread one over the other—in order that the blood will stay there for a long time, so that it is cocted and refined before it flows from it into the ventricles of the brain. *De usu partium* 9.[83]

(44) The spinal cord—in effect, the soft substance which emerges from the brain and runs down the entire spinal vertebrae—is surrounded by exactly the same two membranes as those surrounding the brain. One membrane adheres to the other, and both are surrounded by a third tunic that is coiled around them from the outside just like a third membrane—strong, hard, and sinewy—to protect [the spinal cord] because of its intense, vigorous, and strenuous movement. *De usu partium* 13.[84]

(45) The senses of taste and touch in the tongue originate from one and the same nerve—namely, from that nerve that comes from the third pair of nerves of the brain. It often happens that the sense of taste is harmed, while such a harmful disturbance does not occur to the sense of touch of the tongue, for the sense of taste requires a more exact discrimination.[85] *De locis affectis* 4.[86]

(46) The higher the position of a part of the spinal cord, the more prominent it is; and the danger [of severe damage to the patient] is greater than [in the case of] a part that is lower [in position]. *De locis affectis* 4.[87]

دائمة بدخول الهواء وخروجه. وأمّا العظم الذي يوقّي الدماغ ممّا يلي الوجه والحنك فإنّه مجوّف وأهل التشريح يسمّونه المصفاة. وليس أثقابه مستقيمة كأثقاب المصفاة فإنّ ثقبه مختلفة المجاري بمنزلة الأسفنجة لكيما إذا كان الهواء مفرط البرد ثمّ استنشق لم يكن دخوله إلى بطون الدماغ على استقامة. ثامنة المنافع.

٤٣ . بين عظم أعلى الحنك وبين غشاء الدماغ الصلب الشبكة المنتسجة من العروق الضوارب. وهي تستبطن تحت الدماغ كلّه إلا اليسير منه. وهذه الشبكة طبقات كثيرة كما لو توهّمت شباك كثيرة من شباك الصيّادين مبسوطة بعضها على بعض كي يطول مقام الدم هناك حتى ينضج ويلطف ويخرج لبطون الدماغ. تاسعة المنافع.

٤٤ . النخاع أعني الجرم اللّين الذي يخرج من الدماغ في خرز الصلب كلّها يحيط به تلك الغشاآن بعينهما المحيطان بالدماغ. وأحد الغشائين لازق بالآخر ويحيط بهما صفاق ملفوف عليهما من ظاهرهما بمنزلة غشاء ثالث قوي صلب من جنس العصب ليقيه لشدّة حركته وقوّتها وصعوبتها. ثالث عشر المنافع.

٤٥ . حسّ الذوق وحسّ اللمس في اللسان من عصب واحد بعينه وهو الذي يأتي من الزوج الثالث من عصب الدماغ. وإنّما يعرض مرارا كثيرة أن ينضرّ حسّ المذاق ولا يختلّ حسّ لمس اللسان مثل تلك المضرّة من طريق أنّ حسّ المذاق يحتاج إلى معرفة أشدّ استقصاء. رابعة التعرّف.

٤٦ . كلّ ما كان من أجزاء النخاع أرفع موضعا فهو أشرف وأجلّ خطرا ممّا كان أجلّ سفلا. رابعة التعرّف.

---

٢ وليس أثقابه كأثقاب المصفاة] om. B || ٧ مبسوطة] متوسطة SG || ٨ ويخرج لبطون الدماغ] om. L || ٩– ١٢ النخاع . . . ثالث عشر المنافع] om. L | ٩ وقوّتها] وقوّتهما G || ١٤ ينضرّ (βλάπτεται)] يتغيّر SG : يختلّ L || ١٦ معرفة] معونة B || ١٨ أجلّ] أشدّ EL | ١٨ سفلا] تسفلا BP

(47) The most important organ of speech is the tongue, while the most important organ of the voice is the larynx, next to the muscle which moves it and the nerve that conducts the power from the brain to that muscle. *De locis affectis* 4.[88]

(48) The inner part of the grapelike tunic [of the eye] has soft and moist hairs so that its [manner of] touching the crystalline humor is like touching with a [soaked] sponge. A fine humor—namely, the albuminoid humor—has been made to pour over the crystalline humor in order to form a barrier between the parts of the hornlike tunic that are opposite the perforations of the grapelike tunic and the crystalline and arachnoid tunics. [The albuminoid humor] is smooth as a mirror as it covers the crystalline humor on the outside above the vitreous humor. *De usu partium* 10.[89]

(49) If the membranes surrounding the brain were severed—and, similarly, if one were to cut into the brain substance itself—it would not cause any harm to a living creature.[90] But if the cut should reach the ventricles of the brain, a living creature would be deprived immediately of all its voluntary movements. *De anatomia vivorum* 2.[91]

The bodily movements of living creatures that can be grasped by the senses are of two [types]: voluntary movements, and the movement of the heart and the arteries. There is [also] a third type of movement—namely, that of the veins, which cannot be grasped by the senses but which I do not need to describe at this point. *De tremore,*[92] *palpitatione, [convulsione, et rigore liber].*[93]

(50) Says Moses: The third movement referred to by him[94] here is explained by him in the third book of his work *De naturalibus facultatibus*—namely, that the veins sometimes move to attract the food and sometimes make the opposite movement to discharge some of the food they contain through exactly the same channel.[95] He has given a lengthy explanation of it in that book.

٤٧ . أشرف آلات الكلام اللسان وأشرف آلات الصوت الحنجرة والعضل المحرّك لها والعصب الذي يؤدّي إلى ذلك العضل القوة من الدماغ. رابعة التعرّف.

٤٨ . باطن الطبقة العنبية له خمل رطب ليّن ليصير لقاؤه الرطوبة الجليدية بمنزلة لقاء الأسفنجة. وجعل رطوبة رقيقة وهي البيضية مصبوبة على الرطوبة الجليدية لتحجب بين ما يوازي من القرنية ثقب العنبية وبين الجليدية والطبقة العنكبوتية. وهي الصقيلة كالمرآة ملبّسة على ما هو من الرطوبة الجليدية خارجا ناتئا عن الرطوبة الزجاجية. عاشرة المنافع.

٤٩ . إذا قطعت الأغشية المحيطة بالدماغ وكذلك لو أنّك قطعت من جرم الدماغ نفسه لم يضرّ ذلك بالحيوان في شيء. فأمّا متى بلغ القطع إلى بطونه فإنّ ذلك يسلب الحيوان على المكان جميع الحركات الإرادية. في ثانية تشريح الأحياء.

الحركات التي يدركها الحسّ من حركات أبدان الحيوان حركتان: الحركات الإرادية وحركة القلب والعروق الضوارب. وهنا جنس ثالث من أجناس الحركات يكون في العروق الغير ضوارب لا يدركه الحسّ وليس بي إلى ذكر هذا الجنس في هذا الموضع حاجة. في مقالته في الرعدة والاختلاج.

٥٠ . قال موسى: هذه الحركة الثالثة التي أشار إليها هنا هي التي بيّنها في المقالة الثالثة من كتابه في القوى الطبيعية وهي أنّ العروق الغير ضوارب تارة تتحرّك لجذب الغذاء وتارة تتحرّك ضدّ تلك الحركة لدفع شيء ممّا فيها في تلك الطريق بعينها. وقد طوّل هناك في بيان ذلك.

---

٤ وجعل] وجعلت L | مصبوبة] مصبوغة B || ٥–٦ لتحجب . . . الجليدية] om. L || ٦ الصقيلة] الصقلة SG || ٧ ناتئا] ناتي SGB || ٩–١٠ في شيء . . . الحيوان] om. L || ٩ شيء] من حركاته add. E || ١٠ الأحياء] الأحشاء G || ١٧ تتحرّك ضدّ] تضطرّ L

(51) When we find that the uterus, the stomach, and the gallbladder all attract and discharge through one and the same canal,[96] we should not be surprised that nature often discharges bodily superfluities into the stomach through the veins. Still less [should we be surprised][97] that the stomach is able to attract food from the liver through the same veins by which the food was carried to the liver—namely, during a long [period of] fasting. For if the food canal[98] contains much food, the veins[99] between the liver and the [other] sides of the stomach discharge the food to the liver, and when the food canal[100] is empty and in need of food, it again attracts the food from the liver through the very same veins. *De naturalibus facultatibus* 3.[101]

(52) Locomotion [consists] of firm support and movement. The feet are the instrument of firm support while the thighs and hips are the instrument of movement. *De usu partium* 3.[102]

(53) Of the two ventricles of the heart, the right ventricle was [specifically] created for the sake of the lung, which is the instrument of respiration and [of the] voice. Every living creature that does not inhale the air through its nostrils and mouth has neither a lung nor a right heart ventricle. *De usu partium* 6.[103]

(54) The shape of the stomach is round and elongated, [but] where it approaches the spinal column it flattens against it.[104] In a human being, its lower end is broader than its upper end. The liver surrounds the stomach and is closely clasped by its lobes, just like something that is clasped by the fingers. The spleen touches it on the left side. The lower end of the stomach extends to the right side; behind it is the spinal column and the muscles stretched over it. At its front is a membrane of fat[105] that totally surrounds the stomach to keep it warm. *De usu partium* 4.[106]

٥١ . إذا وجدنا الرحم والمعدة والمرارة كلّها تجذب وتدفع بعنق واحدة بعينها فليس من العجب أن تكون الطبيعة كثيرا ما تدفع إلى المعدة في العروق فضول البدن . وأكثر من ذلك أنّ المعدة يمكن أن تجذب إليها الغذاء من الكبد بالعروق التي حملت منها الغذاء إلى الكبد ويكون ذلك وقت الصوم الطويل . وذلك أنّ العروق الواسطة بين الكبد وسائر نواحي المعدة متى كان في المعدة وما يتّصل بها غذاء كثير نفّذته تلك العروق إلى الكبد وإذا تفرّغت المعدة واحتاجت إلى غذاء جذبته من الكبد ثانية بتلك العروق بأعيانها . في ثالثة القوى .

٥٢ . المشي يتمّ بالثبات والنقلة . والقدمان هما آلة الثبات والساقان والفخذان آلة الحركة . ثالثة المنافع .

٥٣ . التجويف الأيمن من تجويفي القلب إنّما خلق لمكان الرئة والرئة آلة التنفّس والصوت . وكلّ حيوان لا يستنشق الهواء بمنخريه وفمه فهو عديم الرئة وعديم التجويف الأيمن من تجويفي القلب . سادسة المنافع .

٥٤ . شكل المعدة مستديرة متطاولة وهي ممّا يلي الصلب مسطوحة . وأسفلها في الإنسان أوسع من أعلاها . والكبد تحتوي عليها وتلزمها بزوائدها كما يمسك الشيء بالأصابع ، ويلقاها الطحال من الجانب الأيسر . وأسفل المعدة ذاهب نحو الجانب الأيمن ، ومن خلفها الصلب والعضل الممدود عليه . ومن قدّامها غشاء الثرب وهو يلتفّ على المعدة كلّها ليسخنها . رابعة المنافع .

---

٤ الواسطة] الواصلة L || ٥ بين] من G || ٨ آلة] آلات EB || ٩ آلة] آلات EB ||
١٠ لمكان] كون add. EL : بين add. B | والرئة] om. EL

(55) The [membrane of] fat is composed of two dense, fine layers, one lying upon the other, and of arteries, veins, and not a small amount of fat. We do not find in the body of a living creature a membrane that is denser and lighter. *De usu partium* 4.[107]

(56) There is a membrane over the stomach surrounding its exterior, fleshy layer, and this membrane[108] attaches it to the spinal column. The membrane of fat originates from this membrane; likewise, the membrane that covers the liver binds it [to all the inward parts] and surrounds it as a protective skin originates from it. From it, too, originate the membranes of the spleen, urinary bladder, kidneys, and intestines. *De usu partium* 4.[109]

The stomach and intestines are nourished by two things: the first thing is the food that passes through them and is digested in them; and the second thing is that which they attract from the liver. *De usu partium* 4.[110]

(57) After the stomach is filled with an adequate amount of nourishment, it stores the best part of it up in its own layers, and then it expels as residues the remaining amount, which is too much for its nature. Each of the intestines functions in the same way. *De naturalibus facultatibus* 3.[111]

(58) Imagine the whole economy of nutrition divided into three periods. Imagine that in the first period, the nutriment remains in the stomach so that it can be cocted and is then passed to[112] the substance of the stomach until it is satiated from [the nourishment]. Simultaneously, a portion of [the cocted nutriment] rises to the liver. In the second period, it passes along the intestines and is passed to their layers and to the substance of the liver. In this period, a [small] part of it is carried all over the body. Imagine that in this period, that which was passed to the substance of the stomach in the first period is now adherent and attached to it.

٥٥ . الثرب مؤلف من طبقتين كثيفتين رقيقتين إحداهما مطبقة على الأخرى ومن عروق ضوارب وغير ضوارب وشحم ليس باليسير . ولا نجد في بدن الحيوان أكثف وأخف من الغشاء . رابعة المنافع .

٥٦ . على المعدة غشاء يحيط بطبقتها اللحمية الخارجة وهذا الغشاء يربطها مع الصلب . ومن هذا الغشاء غشاء الثرب ومنه ينشأ الغشاء الذي يغشى الكبد ويربطها ويحيط بها وهو لها كالجلد ليقيها . ومنه أيضا تنشأ أغشية الطحال والمثانة والكلى والأمعاء . رابعة المنافع .

المعدة والأمعاء تغتذي بشيئين : أحدهما الغذاء الذي يمرّ بهما وينهضم فيهما والآخر ما تجذبه من الكبد . رابعة المنافع .

٥٧ . المعدة بعد أن تمتلئ من الأطعمة بالمقدار الكافي وتضمّ إلى طبقاتها أجود ما فيه وتزيده عليها بدفع ما يبقى بعد ذلك عنها بمنزلة ثقل خارج في مقداره عن طبعها . وكذلك يفعل كلّ واحد من الأمعاء . في ثالثة القوى .

٥٨ . قسّم في ذهنك تدبير الغذاء إلى ثلاثة أوقات . توهّمه في الوقت الأوّل لابثا في المعدة ليقبل النضج ويزيد في جرم المعدة حتى تشبع منه . وفي هذا الوقت أيضا يرتقي منه شيء إلى الكبد . الوقت الثاني هو عند ما يجوز في الأمعاء ويزيد في طبقاتها وفي جوهر الكبد . ويسير منه أيضا في هذا الوقت شيء يسير إلى البدن كلّه . وتوهّم في هذا الوقت أنّ الشيء الذي زاد في جرم المعدة في الوقت الأوّل قد

---

١ رقيقتين] om. EL || ٢ بدن] أبدان EL || ٥ غشاء] ينشو L : ينشي E || ٦–٧ ويحيط . . . رابعة المنافع] om. E | ٦ لها] om. B || ١١ بدفع] تدفع SP : وتدفع L || ١٣ توهّمه] متوهّمة EL | في] om. EL || ١٤ ويسير] ويصير EL

In the third period, imagine that the stomach receives nutriment by assimilating with its substance that which had become adherent to it in the second period. At the same time, in the intestines and the liver, that which was passed to their substance [before] now becomes adherent and attached to it, while the rest passes to all the other parts of the body and is added to it. *De naturalibus facultatibus* 3.[113]

(59) The digestion that takes place in the stomach is a kind of alteration. The same holds true for the digestion that takes place in the veins and the digestion [that takes place] in every single organ. After this third alteration, there is a fourth alteration called assimilation; and, although this name is different from that of nutrition, their meaning is the same. *De [morborum] causis et symptomatibus* 6.[114]

(60) The omentum[115] is an organ that is not necessary for life to exist; its usefulness for the body is slight. However, since veins and arteries are woven into it, we have become careful not to cut something away from it. If a hemorrhage appears in it, it should be tied off from above and then one may excise [that spot]. *De methodo medendi* 6.[116]

(61) The parenchyma[117] of the spleen is loose, porous, and light like a sponge. It contains many large arteries in order to heat it, so that it can break up the coarse humor that it attracts, and so that there can be cleansed from it the vaporous superfluity which originates in it because of the bad and coarse humor streaming through it. *De usu partium* 4.[118]

(62) The right kidney lies so high that, in some living beings, it reaches up to the liver.[119] The left kidney lies lower, so that the one does not hinder the other in its attraction, as would be the case if they lay on one line.[120] *De usu partium* 4.[121]

(63) The urinary bladder and the gallbladder are reached by vessels that nourish them, apart from the two vessels through which they attract the residue—because the residue reaches them both—in an absolutely pure state without any admixture. And, in particular, the neck of the

التصق واتّصل بجرمها . والجزء الثالث من هذا الزمان تتوهّم المعدة فيه تغتذي بأن تشبه بجرمها ما قد التصق في الوقت الثاني . وأمّا الأمعاء والكبد في هذا الوقت فيلتصق ويتّصل ما زاد في جرمها وينفذ البقية إلى جميع البدن ويزيد فيه . في ثالثة القوى .

٥٩ . الانهضام الذي يكون في المعدة هو نوع من أنواع التغيّر . والانهضام الذي يكون في العروق هو أيضا نوع من أنواع التغيّر وكذلك أيضا الانهضام الذي يكون في كلّ واحد من الأعضاء . وبعد هذا التغيّر الثالث تغيّر آخر رابع يقال له التشبّه واسم التشبّه غير اسم الإغتذاء ومعناهما واحد . في سادسة العلل والأعراض .

٦٠ . الثرب من الأعضاء التي ليست باضطرارية في وجود الحياة ، ومنفعته في البدن يسيرة . لكنّ لمّا انتسجت فيه عروق ضوارب وغير ضوارب صرنا نحذر من قطع شيء منه . إن برز من انبثاق الدم فيربط من فوق وحينئذ يقطع ما برز . سادسة الحيلة .

٦١ . جرم الطحال رخو متخلخل سخيف شبيه بالأسفنج . وفيه عروق ضوارب كثيرة عظيمة لتسخنه حتى يهضم الخلط الغليظ الذي يجذبه ولتنقي منه الفضلة الدخانية المتولّدة فيه لرداءة الخلط الذي يسلك فيه وغلظه . رابعة المنافع .

٦٢ . الكلية اليمنى مرتفعة حتى أنّها في بعض الحيوان تلقى الكبد . والكلية اليسرى أسفل حتى لا تعيق إحداهما الأخرى عن الجذب لو كانتا على سمت واحد . رابعة المنافع .

٦٣ . المثانة وكيس المرار يأتيهما عروق تغذوهما سوى العرقين الذين يجذبان بهما الفضل لأنّ الفضلة تأتيهما وهي خالصة محضة لا يخالطها شيء . ويأتي عنق المرار

---

١ التصق] التزق ELBP | يلتصق] يلتزق ELBP || ٢ التصق] التزق ELBP | والجزء] والوقت EL || ٨ الحياة] الحيوة SE : حيوته L || ١٠ من قطع شيء] ألا نقطع شيئا L : أن نقطع شيء E || ١٣ يهضم] ينهضم SP : ينضج EL || ١٥ الكلية . . . واحد] om. E || ١٦ أحدهما] أحداهما L | كانتا على سمت واحد] كانت أعلى L

gallbladder is reached by an artery, a vein, and a nerve, while each of these is endlessly divided [throughout] the entire body of the gallbladder, and even so the urinary bladder [has a similar ramification of vessels]. *De usu partium* 5.[122]

(64) The uterus has the nature of a nerve and is hard.[123] Women have been created with two uteri that end up in one beginning point—namely, the neck of the uterus.[124] The body of the uterus is covered by an external membrane which joins [the two uteri] together in one place, connects what is between them, and ties them together. [Women] have been created with two breasts, each one like a servant for its half of the uterus.[125] One of the marvels of creation is that [in a woman] the number of uterine cavities is equal to the number of breasts, whereas in other living creatures the number of breasts is equal to the number of offspring. *De usu partium* 14.[126]

(65) The urinary bladder and the uteri are not different with regard to their location. The bladder is harder and more sinewy,[127] however, and therefore, inflammations occurring in it make the pulse harder than uterine inflammations. *De pulsu* 16.[128]

(66) Four organs have two membranes—namely, the esophagus, the stomach, all the intestines, and all the arteries except for those in the lungs. Four organs have only one membrane—namely, the gallbladder, the urinary bladder, the uterus, and all the veins except for the veins in the lungs. *De naturalibus facultatibus* 1 and 3; *De usu partium* 6.[129]

(67) The penis grows out from the pubic bones, from their upper parts, as the other ligaments. But, unlike the [other] ligaments, it has been endowed with a cavity so that it can fill rapidly, empty rapidly, become tensed and hard and then become shrunken and relaxed. This hollow nerve (if you wish, you may call it a "nerve" or give it another name)—I mean, the penis—is embedded far from the anus, and the channel for the semen extends longitudinally in its lower parts and is centrally located. *De usu partium* 15.[130]

(68) There are nerves in the membrane of the two kidneys similar to the nerves of the spleen, liver, and gallbladder; for all these organs receive small nerves that are all connected to the membranes covering them from the outside. But the urinary bladder receives large nerves, so that its sensation is finer and more intense. All these organs are covered by membranes originating from the membrane stretched over the stomach.[131] *De usu partium* 5.[132]

خاصّة عرق ضارب وغير ضارب وعصبة ولا يزال كلّ واحد منها ينقسم في جرم المرارة بأسرها وكذلك المثانة. في خامسة منافع الأعضاء.

٦٤. الرحم من طبيعة العصب وهو صلب. وجعل للمرأة رحمان ينتهيان إلى مبدأ واحد وهو عنق الرحم. ويغشى جرم الرحم غشاء يعلوه من خارج يجمع الرحمين إلى موضع واحد ويصل ما بينهما ويربطهما. وجعل لها ثديان كلّ ثدي بمنزلة الخادم للرحم الذي في شقّه. ومن الأشياء العجيبة في الخلقة مساواة عدد تجويفات الأرحام لعدد الأثداء ⟨و⟩في سائر الحيوان [و]مساواة أثدائه لعدد أولاده. في رابعة عشر المنافع.

٦٥. المثانة والأرحام لا فرق بينهما في الوضع. لكنّ المثانة أصلب وأقرب من جنس العصب. ولهذا كان أورامها أشدّ تصليبا للنبض من أورام الأرحام. سادسة عشر النبض.

٦٦. أربعة أعضاء هي التي هي ذات طبقتين وهي المرئ والمعدة والأمعاء كلّها والعروق الضوارب كلّها إلا ما كان منها في الرئة خاصّة. وأربعة أعضاء هي ذات طبقة طبقة وهي كيس المرارة والمثانة والرحم والعروق الغير ضاربة كلّها إلا ما كان منها في الرئة خاصّة. في الأولى والثالثة من القوى الطبيعية وفي السادسة من منافع الأعضاء.

٦٧. منشأ الإحليل من عظام العانة من أعالي هذه العظام كسائر الرباطات. وخصّ دون الرباطات بالتجويف ليمتلئ سريعا ويستفرغ سريعا ويتوتّر ويصلب ثمّ يذبل ويرتخي. وهذه العصبة الجوفاء إن شئت أن تسمّيها عصبة أو باسم آخر أعني الإحليل مغرّزة بعيد من الدبر ومجرى المني فيه ممّا يلي الجانب الأسفل ممدود بالطول في وسطه. خامسة عشر المنافع.

---

٥ لها] لهما G : له L || ٦ شقّه] شقّته S || ١١ والأمعاء] والمعاء G || ١٣ طبقة] واحدة add. S^2 || ١٥ أعالي] أعلى L || ١٧ يذبل] يدخل L | الجوفاء] المجوفة EL || ١٨ مغرّزة (ἀφεστήξεται)] مجراه L : مجراها E : ومجراه B

(69) The humors that coagulate and form an obstruction in the very solid organs[133] cause a pain stronger than the pain they cause in those organs that are opposite to these organs [in solidity]. The reason is that these last organs stretch more, and the severity of the pain follows the [intensity] of the stretching. Therefore, pains in the urinary bladder are stronger than uterine pains, although the nerves found in both these organs are equal. *De pulsu* 16.[134]

(70) When the muscles of the arms,[135] legs, and face stretch, they become convex; because of the hardness of the bones[136] beneath them, they become convex[137] when they contract toward their middle.[138] When they relax and extend, they flatten. But something happens to the muscles of the chest and abdomen which is opposite to [that which happens to] the muscles of the arms and legs—namely, when they stretch they flatten, because below them are soft organs[139] that sink when these muscles stretch. Consequently, the swelling [of these muscles] is hidden in low places, but when these muscles relax they become convex because then their protrusion becomes more visible. *De motu musculorum* 1.[140]

(71) The movements of all muscles have one aspect [in common]—namely, contraction [and gathering] to their origin. However, movements of various sorts, like those of arms and head, take place through [the use of] many muscles. Each such movement is accomplished by different muscles. *De motu musculorum* 1.[141]

٦٨ . في غشاء الكليتين عصبة مثل عصب الطحال والكبد والمرارة. فإنّ جميع هذه الأعضاء إنّما يأتيها أعصاب صغار تتّصل كلّها بالأغشية المجلّلة عليها من خارج. وأمّا المثانة فيأتيها أعصاب كبار ليكون حسّها ألطف وأبلغ. وجميع هذه الأعضاء موقّاة بأغشية تنبت من الغشى الممدود على البطن. خامسة المنافع.

٦٩ . الرطوبات التي تلحج وتسدّد في الأجسام التي هي أشدّ تلزّزا تحدث من الوجع أشدّ ممّا تحدثه في الأعضاء التي هي ضدّ هذه الأعضاء. لأنّ تلك تتمدّد أكثر ويتبع التمدّد عظم الوجع. ولذلك كانت أوجاع المثانة أشدّ من أوجاع الأرحام وإن كان العصب موجودا في هاذين العضوين بالسواء. سادسة عشر النبض.

٧٠ . العضل الذي في اليدين والرجلين والوجه إذا توتّر يحدودب لصلابة العظام التي تحته ينتأوا عند اجتماعه لوسطه. وإذا استرخى وانبسط يلطى. وعرض لعضل الصدر والبطن شيء مضادّ لعضل اليدين والرجلين وذلك أنّه إذا توتّر لطي لأنّه يجد تحته أجساما ليّنة تنخفض له حين توتّره. فيخفى الاحديداب في المواضع المتطامنة وإذا استرخى احدودب لأنّه يظهر نتوءه ويبرز. في الأولى من كتاب حركات العضل.

٧١ . لحركات جميع العضل جهة واحدة وهي التقلّص والاجتماع الى مبدئه. وإنّما تحدث الحركات المتقنّنة كحركات اليد والرأس بعضل كثيرة. كلّ حركة من تلك الحركات تتمّ بعضلة غير الأخرى. في تلك المقالة.

---

٢ المجلّلة] المدلّلة L : المدلية E(?) || ٣ أعصاب] عصب GP || ٦ تلك] الأعضاء .add EL || ٨ النبض] المنافع EL || ٩ يحدودب] عظم EL : عظام L[1] | العظام] الأعضاء EL || ١٠ ينتأوا] om. EL | لعضل] وأمّا عضل EL | شيء] فـ- EL | إذا] لينه add. B || ١٢ لأنّه] فإنّه B | ليّنة] في المواضع المتضامنة B | تنخفض] تنخفظ SG | الاحديداب] الاحدوداب SP : الاحدواب B || ١٣ احدودب] احدوب BP | نتوءه] توتره S || ١٦ المتقنّنة] المتقلّبة G | بعضل] بعضلات EL

(72) The faculty in the sperm and the faculty that forms out of blood—material suitable for making bones and material suitable for making nerves, and similarly the other materials [suitable for forming] the homogeneous[142] parts—is called the procreative faculty, because it gives birth to and generates material that was not there previously; it is also called the alterative faculty. And the faculty that gives shape to that material so that it can make a certain bone with a certain size and form, and similarly the other homogeneous parts, is called the formative faculty. This faculty has a rational[143] principle, different from the natural principles. The faculty that causes a small bone or nerve to grow, so that it increases in size and bulk, is called the faculty of growth; and the faculty that feeds the organs so that they grow or replaces what has been used up by them, is the nutritive faculty. This faculty accomplishes its function by means of four [other] faculties—namely, the attractive, retentive, [second] alterative, and excretory faculties. The [second] alterative faculty, which is [also] called the digestive [faculty], achieves its end only by means of the powers of adhesion and assimilation. *De naturalibus facultatibus* 1.[144]

(73) The procreative and formative faculties are the dominant ones as long as the fetus is in the uterus, while the nutritive faculty and the faculty of growth are like handmaids to them. After [one's] birth, the formative faculty ceases its activity and the faculty of growth dominates until the end of adolescence, while the nutritive faculty and the alterative or procreative faculty are like assistants and handmaids to [it]. After the end of adolescence, the faculty of growth and the alterative faculty cease activity, while the nutritive faculty remains [active] until the end of one's life. *De naturalibus facultatibus* 1.[145]

(74) The fibers within each of the intestines are circular and are altogether intertwined in its two layers widthwise, for the intestines merely surround and hold their contents and do not attract anything. As for the stomach, some of its fibers are stretched lengthwise because they attract [food], while other fibers are stretched widthwise because they reject [food]. *De naturalibus facultatibus* 3.[146]

◆

٧٢ . القـوة التـي في المني والتي بها يوجد من الدم مـادّة تصلح لتكون عظاما ومادّه تصلح أن تكون عصبا وكذلك سائر موادّ الأعضاء المتشابهة الأجزاء هي التي تسـمّى القوة المولّدة لأنّها تولد وتوجد مادّة لم تكن قبل موجودة وهي تسـمّى أيضا القوة المغيّرة. والقوة التي تشـكّل تلك المادّة حتى تجعل هذا العظم بقدر كذا وبصورة كذا وكذلك في سـائر المتشـابهة الأجزاء هي التي تسمّى القوة المصوّرة. وهي التي لهـا مبدأ آخر عقلي غير المبـادئ الطبيعية. والقوة التي تنمي ذلك العظم الصغير أو العصبة الصغيرة حتى تكبر وتعظم هي التي تسـمّى القـوة المنمية والقوة التي تغذّي العضـو حتى تنمي أو تخلف عليه ما تحلّل منه هي القـوة الغاذية. وتتمّ بأربع قوى جاذبة وماسـكة ومغيّرة ودافعة. وتلك القوة المغيّرة وهي التي تسمّى الهاضمة لا تتمّ غايتها إلا بقوة ملصقة وبقوة مشبهة. في أولى من القوى الطبيعية.

٧٣ . طال ما الجنين في الرحم تكون القوة المولّدة والمصوّرة هما الغالبتان وتكون القوة الغاذية والمنمية كالخادمتين لهما . ومن بعد الولادة تبطل القوة المصوّرة وإلى منتهى الشباب تغلب القوة المنمية وتكون القوة الغاذية والقوة المغيّرة وهي المولّدة كالعونين لهما وكالخادمتين. ومن بعد انتهاء الشـباب تبطل المنميـة والمغيّرة تلك وتبقى الغاذية إلى آخر العمر. في الأولى من القوى.

٧٤ . الشظايا في كلّ واحد من الأمعاء مستديرة تلتفّ عرضا في طبقتيه جميعا لأنّ الأمعاء إنّما تحتوي على ما فيها فقط وتضمّه وليس تجتذب شـيئا من الأشـياء . وأمّا المعدة فبعض الشـظايا التي فيها يمتدّ طولا بسـبب الجذب وبعضها يمتدّ عرضا بسبب العصر. في ثالثة القوى. تمّت المقالة الأولى.

---

٧ تغذّي] تغذو SP || ٨ عليه] عوض add. EL || ٩ ملصقة] ملزقة ELBP || ١١ طال] طـول EL || ١٣ كالعونـين] كالمعينتـين EL || ١٦ طبقتيـه] طبقتـين EL || ١٩ تمّت المقالة الأولى] om. B | الأولى] بعون الله وعدد فصولها سبعون (سبعين E) فصلا add. EL : والحمد

In the name of God, the Merciful, the Compassionate
O Lord, make [our task] easy

The Second Treatise

Containing aphorisms concerning the humors

(1) Blood is something composed of all the humors according to a natural ratio. It is called "blood" because of its dominance over the other humors. And this is what comes out through venesection and cupping. When we say that the body contains four humors—blood, phlegm, yellow bile, and black bile—by blood we do not mean something composed of all the humors, but something existing, in our conception, unmixed with the other humors.[1] *In Hippocratis Epidemiarum* 2.4.[2]

(2) Just as milk contains a watery fluid that is, as it were, the extraction[3] of the thick part, so, too, all humors contain a fine watery fluid. This fluid differs [from the other fluids] according to the nature of the humor

بسم الله الرحمن الرحيم ربّ يسّر

المقالة الثانية

تشتمل على فصول تتعلّق بالأخلاط

١ . الدم هو الشيء المركّب من جميع الأخلاط على المناسبة الطبيعية . وتسمّى باسم الدم لغلبة الدم واستيلائه على الأخلاط الآخر . وهذا هو الذي يخرج بالفصد والحجامة . وإذا قلنا إنّ في البدن أربعة أخلاط الدم والبلغم والمرّة الصفراء والسوداء فليس نعني حينئذ بقولنا الدم الشيء المركّب من جميع الأخلاط لكنّا نعني الشيء الذي يوجد بالوهم غير مخالط لغيره من الأخلاط . في رابعة شرحه لثانية ابيديميا .

٢ . كما يوجد في اللبن رطوبة مائية كأنّها غسالة الجزء الغليظ الذي فيه كذلك يوجد في جميع الأخلاط رطوبة مائية رقيقة . فتختلف بحسب طبيعة الخلط التي

للّه add. P : والحمد للّه وحده add. S || ١ بسم الله . . . ربّ يسّر] om. ELB : بسم الله الرحمن الرحيم S : ربّ يسّر P || ٧ بقولنا الدم] بالدم قولنا إنّه S

of which it forms the watery part. The worst of all is the watery fluid of the black bile; less detrimental is the watery fluid of the yellow bile; even less detrimental is the watery fluid of the phlegm; and the warmest and best of all is the watery fluid or juice[4] of the blood. *In Hippocratis Epidemiarum* 6.2.[5]

(3) The yellow bile, whether it is saturated [in color] or not—and similarly when it is extremely heated until it becomes like egg yolk[6]—originates from veins and arteries. Sometimes a green bile originates in the belly which has the color of leek *(Allium porrum)* or the greenness of verdigris *(acrugo acris)* or of finely colored indigo *(indigofera tinctoria). De atra bile.*[7]

(4) The thick and pure red bile is the one some physicians call "egg-yolk-like." Sometimes I have observed that it is more watery and less red; this one in particular is called the "yellow bile." At other times I have observed that it is mixed with fine phlegm or watery fluid. Another type of bile may originate that has the color of leek. This one often originates in the stomach because of foodstuffs that do not accept coction, such as beet *[Beta vulgaris]*, onion *[Allium cepa]*, and leek. Sometimes it originates in the veins because of unnatural heat and then streams toward the stomach or intestines. *In Hippocratis Prognostica commentarius* 2.[8]

(5) Sometimes red bile with the color of red arsenic is discharged by vomiting and is called "arsenic bile." And sometimes a sediment thereof similar to red arsenic is discharged in the urine. *In Hippocratis Epidemiarum* 6.1.[9]

(6) We call every cold, moist humor in the body "phlegm." There are many types of this humor. A very cold type of it causes extremely severe pains and looks like melted glass. This glassy type tastes somewhat sour. Another type that people often spit out or vomit contains noticeable sweetness and is not absolutely cold because of the sweetness. A third type of [this] humor tastes sour when one vomits it and is less cold than the glassy

هي مائيته. فأخبثها مائية المرّة السوداء وأقلّ منها خباثة مائية الصفراء وأقلّ من ذلك مائية البلغم وأسخنها وأطيبها مائية الدم وصديده. في ثانية شرحه لسادسة ابيديميا.

٣. المرّة الصفراء مشبعة كانت أو غير مشبعة وكذلك إذا أفرطت عليها الحرارة حتى صارت كصفرة البيض تتولّد في العروق والشريانات. وأمّا البطن فإنّه يتولّد فيه أحيانا مرّة خضراء كلون الكرّاث وخضرة الزنجار ونيلنجيه اللون رقيقة. في مقالته في المرّة السوداء.

٤. المرار الغليظ الأحمر الناصع هو الذي يسمّيه بعض الأطبّاء الشبيه بمحّ البيض. وربّما رأيته أكثر رطوبة وأقلّ حمرة وهو الذي يسمّى خاصّة المرار الأصفر. وربّما رأيته قد خالطه بلغم لطيف أو رطوبة مائية. وقد يتولّد جنس آخر من المرار لونه كلون الكرّاث. وهذا يتولّد كثيرا في المعدة بسبب أطعمة لم تقبل النضج مثل السلق والبصل والكرّاث. وربّما تولّد في العروق من حرارة خارجة عن الطبع ثمّ ينصبّ إلى المعدة أو إلى المعاء. في لشرحه الثانية تقدمة المعرفة.

٥. قد يخرج بالقيء مرار أحمر في لون الزرنيخ الأحمر وتسمّى المرّة الزرنيخية. وقد يخرج في البول ثفل منه مثل ذلك أيضا. في الأولى من شرحه لسادسة ابيديميا.

٦. كلّ خلط بارد رطب يكون في البدن فنحن نسمّيه بلغما. ولهذا الخلط أصناف كثيرة فصنف منه بارد جدّا يحدث أوجاعا في غاية الشدّة شبيه في منظره بالزجاج المذاب. وهذا الصنف الزجاجي معه شيء من الطعم الحامض. وصنف آخر كثير ما يتنخّعه ويقذفه الناس معه حلاوة محسوسة وليس بخالص البرد من

---

٢ ثانية] ثامنة S ‖ ٧ الأطبّاء] الناس SEBLP | الشبيه] om. EL ‖ ١١ ثمّ] حتى B ‖ ١٢ ينصبّ] انصبّ EL : ينضج B | المعاء] الأمعاء ELBP | في شرحه لثالثة] في شرحه ب E : في ثانية L : في شرحه لثانية BP ‖ ١٥ بلغما] بلغميا E ‖ ١٧ المذاب] الذائب L ‖ ١٨ يتنخّعه] يتنفه (!)B

one but colder than the sweet one. There is also a salty type, and this one originates either from putrefaction [of the humor] or from the salty, watery fluid mixed with it. *De [differentiis] febrium* 2.[10]

(7) When food is cocted in the liver, the residual substance resembling the foam that floats on grape wine is the natural yellow bile, while the residual substance settling [in a manner] similar to the lees of wine[11] is the black bile. This is the case when the body functions in a natural way.[12] But when the body deviates from nature,[13] the yellow bile becomes similar to egg yolk in color and thickness. This happens when, at any time, the bile is burned and roasted because of fiery heat. The other types of bile are, as it were, intermediate between these two. *De naturalibus facultatibus* 2.[14]

(8)[15] When at the end of book 2 of *De naturalibus facultatibus* Galen speaks about [the fact] that nature has not made an organ[16] for evacuating the natural phlegm from the blood, he says: The superfluity that descends from the head cannot be properly called "phlegm," but should be called "coryza" (mucous discharge from the nostrils). And nature has provided for its evacuation from the body, as I will explain in *De usu partium*.[17] I[18] will also explain[19] the device provided by nature to rapidly cleanse the phlegm from the stomach and intestines, for it is the opposite to that [portion of the phlegm] that streams in vessels, because that [phlegm] is useful to the body and, therefore, nature does not have to evacuate it. It is proper for you to understand that when I use the term uncocted for the phlegm that is in the vessels and that has been given by nature the

أجل حلاوته. وصنف ثالث يحسّـــه من يقذفه حامضا وهو أقلّ بردا من الزجاجي وأبــرد من الحلــو. وصنف مالح وذلك يكون إمّا من قبل عفونته وإمّا من قبل رطوبة مائية مالحة خالطته. في ثانية الحمّيات.

٧. إذا انطبخ الغذاء في الكبد فالفضلة الشـبيهة بالزبد الذي يطفو على عصير العنب هو المرّة الصفراء الطبيعية والذي يرســب شـبيه بالدردي هو المرّة السوداء. هــذا إذا كان أمر البدن جاريا على الأمر الطبيعي. أمّــا إذا كان خارجا عن الطبع فإنّ المرّة الصفراء تصير شبيهة بمحّ البيض في اللون والغلظ. إذا عرض في وقت من الأوقات أن يحترق هذا المرار ويشتوي من الحرارة النارية. وأمّا سائر أنواع المرار فكأنّه متوسّط فيما بينهما. في الثانية من القوى الطبيعية.

٨. בזכרו גלינו בסוף המאמר השני מן הכחות הטבעיות כי הליחה הלבנה הטבעית לא שם הטבע מקום לה להנקותה מן הדם אמר ואמנם המותר אשר ירד מן הראש אין מן הנכון שתקרא ליחה לבנה אבל יקרא מותר היורד מן האף. והטבע השגיח לנקותו מן הגוף כמו שנבאר זה בתועלת האברים. וההשתדלות היותר מבואר אשר השתדל הטבע להריק הליחה הלבנה במהירות מן האצטומכה והמעים כי הוא הפך אשר יגר בעורקים יועיל לגוף ועל כן אין צורך בטבע להריקו. ואמר וראוי שתבין ממאמרי באמרי בלתי מבושל בליחה הלבנה אשר בגידים אשר הכינו הטבע לעשות ממנו

---

٢ وصنف] آخر add. EL || ٣ مالحة] om. EL || ٥ يرسب] شيء add. ELB || ٢٨.١٠–٢٩.٢ בזכרו גלינו בסוף... ממנו דם כלל om. BELGPS || ١١ מקום] כלי פ || ١٣ אמר] om. ב || ١٤–١٥ וההשתדלות... השתדל הטבע] ואבאר התחבולה אשר הערים הטבע פ || ١٧ וראוי] ראוי מ

proper disposition that blood can be made from it, it has a meaning that is different from the term uncocted used for the phlegm in the stomach and intestines, for this does not at all have the proper disposition that blood [be made] from it.[20]

(9) The spleen and the gallbladder purify the blood and each of the two attracts from the blood an amount of [yellow] and black bile of such a quantity and quality that if it were to reach the entire body it would be harmful to it. They leave the remainder in it, for [the blood] that is very thick and earthy and that has entirely escaped alteration in the liver is drawn by the spleen into itself. The remainder [of the blood] that is moderately thick and cooked passes to the entire body, for the blood in many parts of the body needs [a certain] thickness. And the same holds true for the yellow bile.[21] *De naturalibus facultatibus* 2.[22]

(10) Just as in the case of the two biles—whereby one part is useful to a living being and is natural,[23] while the other part is unnatural and useless—so, too, is it [in the case of] phlegm. The sweet part of it is useful to a living being because it is natural; [concerning that part] of it that is sour or salty, that part of it that is sour does not accept any of the second digestion[24] in the liver, while the salty part is putrefied. And everything that is not digested in the first digestion, which takes place in the stomach, is not a humor. *De naturalibus facultatibus* 2.[25]

(11) Sometimes a phlegmatic humor or bile accumulates in the stomach. This phlegmatic humor sometimes varies [in quality], because some of it can be sour, salty, sweet, or tasteless. Some of it can also be moist and thin, some can be thick or viscous, and some easily dissolved. The same holds true for the bile: some is red and some yellow. Each of the two types can be more or less red or yellow. This is exclusive of the types of bile originating in the bodies of ill people. *De alimentorum facultatibus* 1.[26]

(12) The nature[27] of yellow bile is hot and dry. The nature of black bile is cold and dry. Blood is hot and moist, while phlegm is cold and moist. Each of these humors often streams into organs while it is pure,

דם בלתי מה שיובן ממאמרי בלתי מבושל בליחה הלבנה אשר תהיה באצטומכה ובמעים כי זה אינו מוכן שיהיה ממנו דם כלל.

٩ . الطحال والمرارة ينقّيان الدم ويجذب كلّ واحد منهما من الدم من المرار والسوداء المقدار في الكيفية والكمّية الذي لو نفذ إلى جميع البدن أضرّ به . وتركان الباقي فيه . وذلك أنّ ما كان منه شديد الغلظ والأرضية وبالجملة ما فات الكبد إحالته يجذبه الطحال إليه . وما بقي منه بعد ذلك ممّا هو معتدل في الغلظ والنضج ينفذ إلى جميع البدن . وذلك أنّ الدم قد يحتاج في أعضاء كثيرة إلى أن يكون فيه غلظ . وكذلك الحال في الصفراء . في تلك المقالة .

١٠ . كما أنّ المرّتين بعضها نافع للحيوان طبيعي وبعضها خارج عن الطبع لا ينتفع به كذلك أيضا البلغم ما كان منه حلو فهو نافع للحيوان لأنّه طبيعي وما كان منه حامضا أو مالحا فالحامض منه لم يقبل شيئا من النضج الثاني الذي يكون في الكبد وأمّا المالح فعفن . وأمّا كلّ ما لم ينضج النضج الأوّل الذي يكون في المعدة فليس هو خلط من الأخلاط . في تلك المقالة .

١١ . المعدة ربّما اجتمع فيها كيموس بلغمي أو مرّة والبلغم . قد يختلف لأنّ منه حامض ومالح وحلو وما لا طعم له يحسّ . ومنه أيضا ما هو رطب رقيق ومنه غليظ ومنه ما هو لزج ومنه ما هو سهل الانحلال والتفرّق . كذلك المرّة منها حمراء ومنها صفراء وكلّ واحد من الصنفين يزيد وينقص في الحمرة والصفرة وذلك سوى أنواع المرّة التي تتولّد في الأبدان المريضة . أولى الأغذية .

١٢ . المرّة الصفراء قوّتها حارّة يابسة والمرّة السوداء قوّتها باردة يابسة والدم حارّ رطب والبلغم بارد رطب وكلّ واحد من هذه الأخلاط كثيرا ما ينصبّ إلى

---

٢ المقدار] بالمقدار ELBP || ٣ منه] G¹ om. S || ١١ لم] لا ELB || ١٤ مرّة] صفرا add. E || ١٥ يحسّ] om. EL || ٢٠ هذه] om. EL

unadulterated, and unmixed.[28] Sometimes, however, one of them streams [into organs while] mixed with another [humor]. *De [morborum] causis et symptomatibus* 2.[29]

These humors are [usually] mixed with one another. We only rarely find one of them pure, not mixed with another. *De [morborum] causis et symptomatibus* 1.[30]

(13) When we speak of "phlegmatic humors," we mean by this all the humors in which moisture and cold dominate their temperament. When we speak of "melancholic humors," we mean by this all those humors in which dryness and cold dominate. The phlegmatic and melancholic humors are of diverse [categories and] types,[31] [as are] the characteristics that differentiate [them] from each other. *De locis affectis* 3.[32]

(14) The difference between black bile and the other melancholic humors which often leave the body through vomiting and diarrhea is that one can taste and smell black bile because it is clearly sour or bitter, or both at the same time, so that flies do not go near to it. If some of it happens to fall on the ground, it has the same effect as very acidic vinegar. Its consistency is thick, and it originates especially in the bodies of ill people. The other melancholic humors cannot be tasted, nor do flies shy away from them, nor do they cause the ground to effervesce.[33] Even though we call the black [humor] that sometimes originates in the bodies of healthy people "black bile," it is not the same as the one which we have described just now. *De atra bile.*[34]

(15) When the melancholic humor, which is similar to turbid blood [with] its sediment—and this humor is extremely thick, just like the lees of wine—is burned through an ardent fever, it causes bubbles on the ground.

الأعضاء محضا صرفا لا يخالطه شـــيء وربّما انصبّـت مختلطة بعضها مع بعض. ثانية العلل والأعراض.

هذه الأخلاط يخالط بعضها بعضا ولا نكاد نجد واحدا منها خالصا لا يخالطه غيره إلا في الندرة. أولى العلل والأعراض.

١٣. متـــى قلنا أخلاط بلغمية نريد به جميع الأخلاط التي الغالب على مزاجها الرطوبة والبرودة. وقولنا أخلاط سوداوية نريد به جميع الأخلاط التي الغالب عليها اليبـــس والبرودة والأخلاط البلغمية والســـوداوية فصولا وأصناف عظيمة يخصّ كلّ واحد منها على حدته. ثالثة التعرّف.

١٤. الفرق بين المرّة الســـوداء وبين ســـائر الكيموسات السود التي تخرج مرارا كثيرة بالقيء والإســـهال هو أنّ المرّة الســـوداء يحسّ منها بالذوق وبالشـــمّ بحموضة ظاهرة أو عفوصة ظاهرة أو بالأمرين جميعا ولا يقربها الذباب. وإذا ألقي منها شيء على الأرض عرض منه مثل ما يعرض من الخلّ الثقيف. ويكون في قوامها غلظ وهي تتولّد في أبدان المرضى خاصّة. وأمّا سائر الكيموسات السود فلا يحسّ منها بطعم ولا ينفر منها الذباب ولا ينفط منه الأرض. وإن كنّا قد نسمّي السوداء التي تتولّد في أبدان الأصحّاء في بعض الأوقات مرّة سوداء فليست هي هذه التي تقدّمت صفتها. في مقالته في المرّة السوداء.

١٥. ما كان من الســـوداء شبيها بعكر الدم وثقله وهو غليظا غاية الغلظ بمنزلة درديّ الشـــراب إن احترق في حمّى محرقة فهو يحدث في الأرض انتفاخا. ويكون

---

٥ بــه] بهـا E ‖ ٧ والأخلاط] وللأخلاط ELP | فصولا] فصـول ELBP ‖ ١١ ظاهرة] om. S ‖ ١٤ ينفر] يفرّ ELBP | ينفط] تغلى EL : تجفظ B | منه] om. B : منها EL ‖ ١٧ وثقله] وفضله G ‖ ١٨ في حمّى] فتسمّي EL

At the same time, it is only very slightly sour or not sour at all. I usually call it "melancholic humor" or "melancholic blood," because it is not proper to call something in this condition "black bile." *De locis affectis* 3.[35]

(16) Diseases caused by black bile are cancer, elephantiasis, mange,[36] the disease in which the skin peels off,[37] quartan fever, delusion,[38] and thickness of the spleen. *De alimentorum facultatibus* 3.[39]

(17) The juice that is called "crude" is like that which one can see as sediment in the urine of someone who suffers from fever due to a surplus of raw phlegms.[40] It also settles in the urine of healthy people—namely, of someone who is tired and then eats hard foods that are difficult to digest. This juice is similar to pus. The difference between them is that the crude juice does not stink and is not sticky, [although] it is similar to [pus] in color and consistency. *De alimentorum facultatibus* 1.[41]

(18) The stomach of a young child's body cannot completely digest what he needs for growth and nutrition. Therefore, the bodies [of young children] draw out the food from their stomachs before it has been thoroughly digested, with the result that [these children] have a large quantity of raw superfluities. *De crisibus* 1.[42]

(19) The humor consisting of yellow bile has a drying effect just like salt water and sea water. For this reason, the membranes of the arteries of someone suffering from jaundice are drier [than normal]. Even if he does not have fever, his pulse becomes harder. *De pulsu* 12.[43]

(20) When the biting humor in the stomach is the type of yellow bile, it rises to the cardia of the stomach because of the lightness of the yellow bile. When this biting humor is like leek or sour or salty, it settles in the cavity of the lining of the stomach[44] and does not rise or ascend to its cardia. *Mayāmir* 2.[45]

مع هذا قليل الحموضة جدّا أو لا يكون حامضا أصلا . ومن عادتي أن أسمّيه خلطا سوداويا أو دما سوداويا لأنّ ما كان في هذا الحدّ لم يستحقّ أن يسمّى مرّة سوداء . ثالثة التعرّف .

١٦ . الأمراض الحادثة عن السوداء السرطان والجذام والجرب والعلّة التي يتقشّر الجلد فيها وحمّى الربع ووسواس وغلظ الطحال . ثالثة الأغذية .

١٧ . الكيموس الذي يقال له الخام هو بمنزلة ما يرى راسبا في بول من يحمّ من قبل كثرة النخم . فيرسب أيضا في بول من يتعب من الأصحّاء ويتناول أغذية صلبة عسرة الانهضام . وهو شبيه بالقيح . والفرق بينهما أنّ الخام ليس بمنتن ولا لزج وهو مثله في اللون والقوام . أولى الإغذية .

١٨ . معدة بدن الصبي لا تفي بهضم ما يحتاج إليه من النشوء والإغتذاء ولذلك تجتذب أبدانهم الغذاء من معدهم من قبل أن يستحكم نضجه فيها فيكثر الفضل النيء فيهم . أولى البحران .

١٩ . من شأن خلط المرّة الصفراء أن يجفّف بمنزلة ما يجفّف الماء المالح وماء البحر . وبهذا السبب تجعل صفاقات عروق صاحب اليرقان أجفّ . وإن كان بلا حمّى فيصير نبضه أصلب وأصغر . ثانية عشر النبض .

٢٠ . الخلط اللذّاع الذي يكون في المعدة متى كان من جنس المرّة الصفراء فبسبب ما هي عليه المرّة الصفراء من الخفّة يتصاعد نحو فم المعدة . ومتى كان هذا الخلط اللذّاع كرّاثيا أو حامضا أو مالحا فإنّه يرسب في تجويف خمل المعدة ولا يرتقي ولا يطفو في فمها . ثانية الميامر .

---

٢ لم] لا EL || ٨ النخم] G(?) : التخم SELBP || ١١ النيء] الذي GB || ١٣ ما يجفّف] om. EL || ١٤ عروق] عرق GBP || ١٧ فبسبب] فلسبب EL

(21) Sometimes a sharp humor descends in the direction of the buttocks and—since it refuses to be expelled—is by necessity retained[46] by the person. This humor then goes back and rises again, causing a burning [pain] in the stomach. It fills the head with vapor that it expels [upward]. In the same way, it often happens that flatulent gas seeking an exit from below [if it is blocked] returns and reascends. *De [morborum] causis et symptomatibus* 6.[47]

(22) If a superfluity streams from [a stronger] organ to a [weaker] organ, it putrefies in that place and becomes [even] worse, and [it] corrupts the food[48] that was brought to [the organ] subsequently, although [the food] was good and useful on its own. *De [morborum] causis et symptomatibus* 2.[49]

(23) Whatever superfluities remain in the body for a long time obviously putrefy, some in a shorter and some in a longer time. When they reach this state, they become pungent and harmful to the organs in which they are retained. This does not happen to the gallbladder, because it possesses [only] a few nerves. But, if the bile becomes a heavy burden to [the gallbladder] because of its large quantity or because of a change in its quality, it becomes pungent and acrid and desires to be expelled. Sometimes the bile is expelled toward the liver through the neck [of the gallbladder] itself, by which it is attracted. *De naturalibus facultatibus* 3.[50]

(24) Constant dyspepsias are extremely strong in producing bad humors and diseases, whether these dyspepsias are due to foods with good chymes or to foods with bad chymes. But dyspepsia caused by bad chymes is much worse than the other one. *De probis malisque [alimentorum] sucis.*[51]

(25) There are two kinds of foods with bad chymes: thin and thick. The bad chyme that is thin causes acute diseases and malignant fevers; and, when it reaches an organ, it causes erysipelas, shingles,[52] and other pains. The thick [bad] chyme causes arthritis, gout, pain in the kidneys, asthma, and hardness of the spleen and liver. When the bad chyme is

٢١. قد ينحدر إلى ناحية الدبر خلط من الأخلاط الحادّة فيحبسه الإنسان ويستكرهه على منعه من الخروج. فيعود الخلط ويصعد ثانيا ويحدث في المعدة لذعا. ويملأ الرأس من البخار الذي يدفعه إليه. وعلى هذا المثال يحدث مرارا كثيرة إذا احتبست الريح التي تطلب الخروج من أسفل فإنّها تعود وترجع إلى فوق. سادسة العلل والأعراض.

٢٢. الفضل إذا انصبّ من عضو إلى الأعضاء يعفن هناك ويزداد شرّا ورداءة ويفسد ما يأتي الأعضاء بعد ذلك من الغذاء وإن كان جيّدا في نفسه نافعا. ثانية العلل والأعراض.

٢٣. الفضول التي تلبث في البدن مدّة طويلة أيّها كان يعفن عفونة بيّنة بعضها في زمان يسير وبعضها في زمان طويل. فإذا صارت بهده الحال لذعت وآذت الأعضاء التي هي فيها محتبسة. وليس يعرض ذلك لكيس المرار لقلّة ما فيه من الأعصاب. ولكنّ إذا ثقل عليه المرار لكثرته أو استحالت كيفيته فصار لذّاعا حرّيفا يتوق حينئذ لدفعه. وقد تدفع المرارة إلى الكبد بالعنق بعينها التي جذبت بها. في ثالثة القوى.

٢٤. التخم المتواترة عظيمة القوة في توليد الكيموس الرديء وتوليد الأمراض سواء كانت التخم من أطعمة حسنة الكيموس أو من أطعمة رديئة الكيموس. إلا أنّ الكائنة من الرديئة الكيموس أشرّ من التخمة الأخرى جدّا. في مقالته في الكيموس الجيّد والرديء.

٢٥. لما كانت الأطعمة الرديئة الكيموس صنفين لطيفة وغليظة. فما كان من الكيموس الرديء لطيفا فهو يحدث أمراضا حادّة وحمّيات خبيثة وإن صار إلى عضو أحدث ورم الحمرة والورم الساعي وآلام غيرها. وما كان منه غليظا فهو يحدث وجع المفاصل والنقرس ووجع الكلى والربو وجساء الطحال والكبد. وما كان مع

---

٢ ويستكرهه على منعه] ويمنعه L || ٤ وترجع] وتصعد EL || ٦ من عضو إلى الأعضاء] إلى عضو من الأعضاء ELBP || ٧ ما] بما B || ١١ أو استحالت] واستحالة L | يتوق] يشوق EL || ١٢ بها] الفضل add. EL

[both] thick and melancholic, it causes cancers, peeling of the skin,[53] itch,[54] quartan fevers, melancholy, a bad complexion,[55] and hemorrhoids. *De probis malisque [alimentorum] sucis.*[56]

(26) Sometimes phlegm occurs with body heat because, when the stomach becomes greatly heated, it cannot digest the food it contains, with the result that the phlegm increases in it. *In Hippocratis De mulierum affectibus commentarius.*[57]

(27) Chymes which dominate in quantity or quality are five: phlegm, yellow bile, black bile, blood, and its watery part. *In Hippocratis Aphorismos commentarius* 1.[58]

(28) Among all the humors, only phlegm does not give rise to black bile, even when it is surrounded by exceedingly strong, burning heat. *In Hippocratis De aere [aquis locis] commentarius* 2.[59]

(29) The superfluity of black bile is the least [abundant] of all the superfluities, the superfluity of yellow bile is more [abundant than the black], and the watery superfluity is many times more [abundant] than [the others]. *De usu partium* 5.[60]

(30) That melancholic humor is natural which does not produce seething and bubbling on the earth when it is poured over it, while that which has taken on this quality is unnatural, because it has assumed a sharpness owing to its burning caused by the unnatural heat. This occurs when the natural melancholic humor putrefies. *De naturalibus facultatibus* 2.[61]

This is the end of the second treatise,
by the grace of God, praise be to Him.

◆

غلظه ذا مرّة سوداء فهو يحدث السرطانات وتقشّر الجلد والحكّة وحمّيات الربع والمالنخوليا وسماجة الوجه والبواسير. في مقالته في الكيموس الجيّد والرديء.

٢٦. قد يعرض البلغم مع حرارة البدن من قبل أنّ المعدة تصير بقوة الحرارة لا تهضم ما يكون فيها من الطعام فيكثر فيها البلغم. في شرحه لأوجاع النساء.

٢٧. الكيموسات التي تغلب بكمّيتها أو بكيفيتها خمسة: البلغم والمرّة الصفراء والمرّة السوداء والدم ومائية الدم. في شرحه للأولى من الفصول.

٢٨. البلغم وحده من بين سائر الأخلاط لا يتولّد منه مرّة سوداء وإن أحاط به حرارة زائدة شديدة محرقة. في شرحه للثانية من الأهوية.

٢٩. الفضلة السوداء أقلّ الفضول كلّها والفضلة الصفراء أكثر من السوداء والفضلة المائية أكثر منها بأضعاف كثيرة. في خامسة منافع الأعضاء.

٣٠. الخلط السوداوي ما لم يحدث منه إذا صبّ على الأرض غليان وانتفاخ فهو طبيعي وما كان قد انتقل إلى هذه الحال فهو خارج عن الطبيعة لأنّه قد استفاد حدّة بسبب احتراقه من الحرارة الخارجة عن الطبيعة. ويحدث هذا عند عفونة الخلط السوداوي الطبيعي. في ثانية القوى الطبيعية. تمّت المقالة الثانية ولله الحمد والمنّة.

---

١ وتقشّر] وتقشير EL ‖ ٢ والمالنخوليا] والمالنخونيا EL | الوجه] اللون E ‖ ٧ البلغم.. .محرقة] فأمّا البلغم وهو وحده من سائر الأخلاط إذا أحاطت به حرارة زائدة شديدة محرقة لم يمكن أن يتولّد منه مرّة سوداء (Galen, *In Hipp. De aere* 3.4.2.09914–09915) ‖ ٨ محرقة] محترقة O ‖ ١٠ منها] منهما L ‖ ١٢ إلى] غير add. EL | هذه] ذلك S | عن] من E ‖ ١٤ السوداوي] وهي add. L | تمّت] كملت EL | ولله الحمد والمنّة] والحمد للّه تعالى وعدد فصولها ثلثين L : عدد فصولها ثلاثون P : والحمد للّه ربّ العالمين كثيرا E : الله أكبر كبيرا add. S

In the name of God, the Merciful, the Compassionate
O Lord, make [our task] easy

The Third Treatise

Containing aphorisms concerning the principles of the art and general rules

(1) The age of adolescence is the one in which the temperament is the best and most balanced. *In Hippocratis De natura hominis commentarius.*

(2) The age between fourteen and twenty-five years is that in which the pubic hair grows.[1] *In Hippocratis Aphorismos commentarius* 5.[2]

(3) The temperament in the age when one is past one's prime[3] and in old age is cold and dry. A clear, defining difference[4] between the age of those who are past their prime and old age is the domination of the moist superfluities [in the latter], along with a clear weakening of all bodily functions. *De marcore.*[5]

بسم اللّه الرحمن الرحيم ربّ يسّر

المقالة الثالثة

تشتمل على فصول تتعلّق بأصول الصناعة وقوانين عامّية

١ . سنّ المراهقين أفضل الأمزاج وأعدلها . في شرحه لطبيعة الإنسان .

٢ . السـنّ التي بين أربعة عشر سنة وبين خمسة وعشرين سنة هي سنّ إنبات الشعر على العانة . في شرحه لخامسة الفصول .

٣ . مزاج سنّ الكهول والشيوخ بارد يابس . والحدّ البيّن الفاصل بين سنّ المكتهلين وبين سنّ الشـيخوخة هي غلبة الفضول الرطبة مع تبيين ضعف جميع أفعال البدن . في مقالته في الذبول .

---

١ بسم اللّه . . . ربّ يسّر] om. ELP : بسم اللّه الرحمن الرحيم S : ربّ يسّر P || ٥ الأمزاج] الأسنان EL || ٦ سنّ] كون B || ٨ البيّن الفاصل بين] الذي بين فصل L : البيّن بين E || ٩ وبين سنّ] وسنّ EL | هي] هو SELBP | ضعف] om. B : في add. L

(4) The whole body of a man breathes well when it is clean and free of superfluities and pressure. The body of a woman has the opposite characteristic, because the spaces between her vessels are narrow on account of the fat, tender flesh and phlegmatic superfluities which occupy them; and, since her skin is thick and firm, hardly anything is dissolved through it.[6] *De pulsu* 11.[7]

(5) The quick dissolution [of humors through perspiration taking place] in the bodies of young people is of great benefit to them and provides quite a few[8] opportunities for the healing of diseases occurring in their bodies, for the improvement of their temperaments when they differ [from their normal state], and for the correction of an abundance and thickness of their humors. *De pulsu* 14.[9]

(6) Porous bodies which are porous are quickly affected by diseases caused by external factors, while [internal] diseases caused by superfluous humors originate in them [only] rarely. In compact bodies, the situation is the reverse. *De optima [corporis nostri] constitutione.*[10]

(7) Bodies with a loose texture[11] are weaker, but their health is more lasting, and when they fall ill they recover quickly. Dense[12] bodies have the opposite characteristics. *In Hippocratis De alimento commentarius* 3.[13]

(8) When an organ is weak, one feels heaviness in it, even when only a small amount [of superfluities] streams toward it. A hot tumor[14] often occurs due to the weakness of an organ, even though the body is not full [of superfluities]. *De [curandi ratione per] venae sectione.*[15]

(9) When the flesh, fat, and chymes in someone's body become more than the previous quantity, while its strength remains the same as before, the movements [of the body] necessarily weaken, since the mover remains the same as before, while those things which are moved became more than their previous quantity. *De plenitudine liber.*[16]

٤ . بدن الرجل كلّه يتنفّس تنفّسا جيّدا وهو نقي معرّى من الفضول ومن الضغط . وبدن المرأة بخلاف هذا وذلك أنّ المواضع التي فيما بين العروق فيها ضيّقة لما يشغلها من الشحم واللحم الرخص والفضول البلغمية والجلد منها كثيف مستحصف عسر ما يتحلّل منه شيء . حادية عشر النبض .

٥ . سرعة تحلّل أبدان الصبيان خير عظيم لهم ليس بيسير الموقع في إصلاح ما يحدث في أبدانهم من المرض وإصلاح مزاجهم المختلف وإصلاح كثرة أخلاطهم وغلظها . رابعة عشر النبض .

٦ . الأجسام المتخلخلة تسرع إليها الأمراض التي أسبابها من خارج ويقلّ فيها تولّد الأمراض التي أسبابها من فضلات الأخلاط . أمّا الأجسام المتلزّزة فالأمر فيها بعكس هذا . في مقالته في أفضل الهيئات .

٧ . الأبدان السخيفة أضعف وأدوم صحّة وإذا مرضت يسهل بروؤها . والأبدان الكثيفة بالضدّ في هذه الأحوال . في شرحه لثالثة الغذاء .

٨ . متى كان بعض الأعضاء ضعيفا أحسّ الإنسان فيه بثقل وإن كان الذي انصبّ إليه يسيرا . وكثيرا ما يحدث الورم الحارّ بسبب ضعف العضو من غير أن يكون البدن ممتلئا . في مقالته في الفصد .

٩ . إذا زاد اللحم والشحم والكيموسات في بدن أحد على المقدار الذي كان وبقيت القوة على حالها الأولى فلا بدّ ضرورة من أن تضعف الحركات إذ المحرّك باقيا على حاله الأولى وقد زادت الأشياء المتحرّكة على المقدار الأوّل . في مقالته في الكثرة .

---

١ الرجل] الرجال SG ‖ ٢ المواضع التي] الموضع الذي S ‖ ٥ أبدان الصبيان] الأبدان التي للصبيان EL ‖ ١١ أضعف] أصعب (!)L (?)E

(10) Most susceptible to spasms are the bodies of children because of the weakness of the body of the nerves[17] in them. Consequently, this affliction occurs to them through the slightest cause, although it is the least dangerous in them. *In Hippocratis Epidemiarum* 1.2.[18]

(11) It is impossible for the strength of an elderly person to be great. Some physicians think that children also do not have great strength, but they are mistaken in their opinion. *De [curandi ratione per] venae sectione.*[19]

As far as the requirement of temperament is concerned, the longest-living people are those whose temperament is the moistest. They are also more able than others to keep their health, and up until the last [stages] of senility [they] have stronger bodies than others who are of the same age. This is [only] on condition that they take care to expel the superfluities from their bodies through exercise, through bathing before taking a meal, through cleansing themselves from their urine and excrements, through purging themselves at times, and through occasionally purifying their heads by means of gargling and chewing, for superfluities originate in the bodies of people with this temperament and those with a warm and moist temperament. *De sanitate tuenda* 6.[20]

(12) The worst of all temperaments is the one that is dry. This is inevitable, since what happens to old people in the course of time is present in them from the very beginning.[21] Sexual intercourse is most harmful [for them] and is contrary to the health of everyone whose temperament tends to dryness. *De sanitate tuenda* 6.[22]

(13) You should know for certain that if a part of the body is full, or has bad humors, or is very sensitive, or if all these attributes occur together, it will undoubtedly form a tumor if an accident[23] should occur to that part, whatever part it is. It is therefore necessary to not seal the place where the

١٠ . أشدّ الأبدان تهيّأ لقبول التشنّج أبدان الصبيان لضعف جسم العصب فيها . ولذلك تسـرع إليهم هذه العلة من أدنى سـبب وهو فيهم أقلّ خطرا . في الثانية من شرحه للأولى من ابيديميا .

١١ . لا يمكن أن تكون قوة من هو في سنّ الشيخوخة قوة شديدة . وقد ظنّ قوم من الأطبّاء أنّ الصبيان أيضا ليس لهم شـدّة من القوة وقد أخطؤوا في هذا الحكم . في مقالته في الفصد .

أطول الناس عمرا بحسـب ما يوجبه المزاج أرطب الناس مزاجا . وهؤلاء أولى من غيرهم بالبقاء على الصحّة ويكونون أقوى بدنا إلى آخر مدّة الهرم من غيرهم ممّن هو في هذه السـنّ . وبشـرط أن يعني بإدرار الفضول من أبدانهم بالرياضة وبدخول الحمّام قبل الطعام وبنفض البول والبراز والإسـهال فـي أوقاته وتنقية الرأس بالغرغرة والمضـوغ في بعـض الأوقات . لأنّ أصحاب هذا المزاج والمـزاج الحارّ الرطب تتولّد الفضول في أبدانهم . سادسة تدبير الصحّة .

١٢ . أردى الأمزجـة كلّها المزاج اليابس . وذلك واجب من قبل أنّ الذي يعرض للمشايخ على طول الزمان هو موجود في هؤلاء منذ أوّل الأمر . والجماع أشدّ الأشياء ضررا ومقاومة للصحّة لكلّ من مزاجه مائل إلى اليبس . سادسة تدبير الصحّة .

١٣ . ينبغي لك أن تعلم علما يقينا أنّ ما كان من الأبدان ممتلئا أو كانت أخلاطه رديئـة أو كان ذكي الحسّ أو كان جامعا لهذه الخلال كلّها فإنّه متى أصابته وجبة في أيّ عضـو كان فلا بدّ أن يحدث له ورما . فلذلـك ينبغي أن لا تلحم موضع القرحة

---

٨ آخـر مـدّة الهـرم] مدّة هذا الهـرم EL || ٩ هذه] هـذا EL || ١٣ يعـرض] om. EL ||
١٧ وجبة] وجع B || ١٨ يهرم] بهرم add. L | تبعته] تتبعه SB يتبعه E

wound[24] might occur, but, rather, to put ingredients on it that soften, alleviate, and allay the pain[25] to prevent the formation of a tumor. *De methodo medendi* 6.[26]

(14) If the substance of someone's heart dries only a little bit, he quickly becomes decrepit but may under [certain] circumstances live for some more years. However, if the substance of someone's heart dries out thoroughly, it will lead to rapid wasting, and he will die shortly. After this [in order of harm] comes the wasting caused by dryness of the liver. Then comes the wasting originating from the stomach when it dries out, and then the wasting originating from other organs. *De methodo medendi* 7.[27]

(15) You should know that if the dryness of the main organs[28] lasts for a long time, it will inevitably be followed by coldness, because the organs are nourished by a hot humor—namely, blood—and, when the organs dry out, their nourishment is cut off and they become dry; this is followed by coldness. *De methodo medendi* 7.[29]

(16) Bodily superfluities are sparse in winter, because the cold congeals them; but in the summer they are plentiful, because the heat melts them.[30] Only a few people combine much food with much drink. *In Hippocratis De aere [aquis locis] commentarius* 1.[31]

(17) Sperm and blood are of one temperament in the winter and of a [different] temperament in the summer. Therefore, the fetuses in these seasons are different, because the summer heat burns and dries the sperm, while the winter cold makes it cold and moist. *In Hippocratis De aere [aquis locis] commentarius* 3.[32]

(18) The rising of the Pleiades [marks] the beginning of summer, and their setting [marks] the beginning of winter. The rising of Virgo[33] [marks] the beginning of autumn, and its setting [marks] the beginning of spring. *In Hippocratis De aere [aquis locis] commentarius* 2.[34]

وتضع عليه الأشياء الملينة المسكنة البعيدة عن أن توجع حتى لا يحدث ورم. سادسة الحيلة.

١٤ . من يبس جرم قلبه يبسا يسيرا فإنّه يهرم سريعا لكنّه على حال يعيش سنينا . أمّا من استحكم يبس جرم قلبه فأمره يؤول إلى الذبول بسرعة ويموت بسرعة. وبعد هذا الذبول الحادث عن يبس الكبد . وبعده الذبول الذي يكون مبدأه من المعدة إذا جفّت وبعده الذبول الذي يبتدئ من أعضاء آخر غير هذه. سابعة الحيلة.

١٥ . ينبغي أن تعلم أنّ يبس الأعضاء الأصلية إذا طالت مدّته تبعته لا محالة برودة لأنّ الأعضاء تغتذي من كيموس حارّ وهو الدم وإذا يبست الأعضاء انحسم غذاؤها وجفّت وتبع ذلك البرد . سابعة الحيلة.

١٦ . فضول البدن في الشتاء قليلة لأنّ البرد يجمّدها وفي الصيف كثيرة لأنّ الحرّ يذيبها وقلّ من يوجد من الناس يجمع كثرة الطعام وكثرة الشراب. في شرحه للأولى من كتاب الأهوية.

١٧ . المني والدم يكونان في الشتاء على مزاج وفي الصيف على مزاج فلذلك تختلف الأجنّة في هذه الأزمنة لأنّ حرارة الصيف تسخن المنّي وتجفّفه وبرد الشتاء يبرده ويرطبه. في شرحه الثالثة للأهوية.

---

٨ تغتذي] تمتلئ SG || ٩ وتبع] ويتبع S || ١٠ فضول . . يذيبها] قال جالينوس إنّ فضول الأبدان تقلّ في الشتاء لأنّ البرد يجمّدها وتكثر في الصيف لإذابة الحرارة لها Galen, *In Hipp. De aere* 1.8.12.02911–02912 || ١١ وقلّ . . . الشراب] وقلّ من يوجد من الناس من يجمع كثرة الطعام والشراب جميعا Galen, *In Hipp. De aere* 1.8.10.02815–09816 | من يوجد من الناس] ما يوجد من الناس من E || ١٣ المني . . . ويرطبه] وذلك أنّ المني والدم يكونان في الشتاء على نوع وفي الصيف على نوع آخر والأجنّة التي تكون في هذه الأزمنة هي مخالفة فنقول الآن إنّ بقرلط لمّا أراد أن يعلمنا أنّ مزاج البلاد في الأزمان كلّها واحد عنى البرودة فقال أنّ مزاج البلاد في الأزمان كلّها واحد عنى البرودة فقال أنّ الأطفال يشبه بعضهم بعضا وذلك أنّه لا يكون عندهم في

(19) Some persons have seen vessels[35] generated in large wounds,[36] as we ourselves have also seen veins that were quite important and numerous[37] in the head and other organs. They do not grow in many people, but only in [a few] individuals, and that rarely.[38] As for arteries and nerves, no one has ever seen them generated, even rarely, in anyone. *De semine* 1.[39]

(20) The empty spaces between the major organs are filled with moisture. This moisture is the nutriment that is especially fit for the homogeneous parts, which they attract from the adjacent parts, but not from the vessels. *De arte parva.*[40]

(21) When the vertebrae of the back separate from each other, there is a white, sticky moisture in the space between them, similar to the moisture that has been poured around the other joints. And equally, around the spinal medulla a sticky humor has been poured similar to the humor that has been poured around the ligament through which the vertebrae of the back are bound together and around all the joints, tongue, and larynx, as well as all the parts that must move continually. *De usu partium* 13.[41]

(22) The tendon is the principal instrument for motion. The muscle was created to produce tendons from it and also to provide the use of composite flesh. Part of the tendon [of the muscles] is connected to the members of hands and feet through its fleshy parts.[42] *De usu partium* 12.[43]

١٨. طلوع الثريّا هو أوّل الصيف وغروبها هو أوّل الشتاء وطلوع السماك هو أوّل الخريف وغروبه هو أوّل الربيع. في شرحه الثانية من الأهوية.

١٩. العروق قد رآها قوم تولّدت في القروح العظيمة كما قد رأيناها نحن أيضا في الرأس وفي أعضاء أخرى تولّدت فيها عروق صالحة في العظم وفي العدد. وليس يتولّد ذلك في خلق كثير لكنّ في الفرد بعد الفرد وفي الندرة. أمّا الشريانات والعصب فلم يرها أحد قط تولّدت في أحد ولو في الندرة. في الأولى من كتابه في المني.

٢٠. المواضع الخالية التي فيما بين الأعضاء الأصلية هي مملوؤة رطوبة. وهذه الرطوبة هي الغذاء الخاصّ للأعضاء المتشابهة الأجزاء التي تجتذبه بالمجاورة لا من العروق. من الصناعة الصغيرة.

٢١. في ما بين خرز الظهر إذا تباعدت بعضها من بعض رطوبة بيضاء لزجة شبيهة بالرطوبة المصبوبة في سائر المفاصل. وعلى النخاع أيضا رطوبة لزجة مصبوبة مثل الرطوبة المصبوبة على الرباط المعقّب به خرز الظهر وفي المفاصل كلّها واللسان والحنجرة وجميع الأعضاء التي تحتاج أن تتحرّك حركات متوالية. ثالثة عشرة المنافع.

٢٢. الوتر آلة أوّلية للحركات. والعضلة خلقت ليكون منها الأوتار ويكون مع هذا ينفع منفعة اللحم المركّب. وبعضه يتّصل بأوصال اليدين والرجلين بأجزائه اللحمية. ثانية عشرة المنافع.

Galen, *In Hipp. De* الصيف حرارة زائدة تحرّق المني وتيبّسه ولا في الشتاء برد مفرط يجمّد المني *aere* 4.5.15.14803–14807 || ١ طلوع . . . الشتاء] . . . وأن يقول إنّ استواء الليل والنهار بعد الشتاء هو أوّل زمان الربيع وإنّ طلوع الثريّا هو أوّل الصيف وغروبها هو أوّل الشتاء فإن كان لم يرد أن يضع استواء الليل والنهار بعد الصيف ويجعله أوّل الخريف فلو قال إنّ طلوع أرقطورس هو أوّل الخريف Galen, *In Hipp. De aere* 2.5.3.08801–08804 || ٤ العدد] الغدد P || ٨ تجتذبه] تغتذي به B || ١٤ للحركات] للحركة EL || ١٥ المركّب] om. SEGLP : وبعض العضل ينتهي إلى وتر واحد عظيم add. B

The nose is the first and foremost instrument of respiration in order.[44] As for the mouth, whatever protection it may provide to a living being against the disasters and calamities that might befall him and force him [to use it for respiration], it is not [primarily] an instrument of respiration. *De usu partium* 11.[45]

(23) There is no other organ in the body with so great an innate property [that enables it] to stretch and extend and then to return and contract into a small space, as the uterus. Since it is attached by means of ligaments to the spine on both sides,[46] these ligaments must also, of necessity, stretch and return to their original state, together with the uterus; they must follow it in its coming and going so that they will be protected from being broken off and [so that] the uterus will be safe and sound. *De usu partium* 14.[47]

(24) The temperament of the [nervous system] is colder than that of any other [organ]. Therefore, it is quickly affected by[48] the cold and conveys to the brain the harm that the cold has inflicted on it. Because of that, one should not approach the place of a nerve, nor touch it with something cold, [and] especially not in the case of abscesses. *De methodo medendi* 6.[49]

(25) The worst city is that which is sheltered from the east winds and in which hot and cold winds blow. *In Hippocratis De aere [aquis locis] commentarius* 1.[50]

(26) A bad temperament harms the faculties [of the body] in their specific essential nature. If the temperament is extremely bad, it annihilates any faculty [of the body]. *De [morborum] causis et symptomatibus* 6.[51]

(27) A varying bad temperament can occur in the whole body, as [in the case of] dropsy of the flesh and in the case of all the fevers except for hectic fever. It can also occur in one part of the body, as [in the case of]

المنخـــران أوّل آلات النفس وأقدمها مرتبة. فأمّا الفم فمهما ســلّم به الحيوان من الآفات والعاهات التي تضطرّه وترهقه فليس هو من آلات التنفّس. حادثة عشر المنافع.

٢٣. ليس في البدن عضو آخر مطبوع على أن يتمدّد ويتّســع اتّساعا كثيرا ثمّ يرجع فيجتمع إلى موضع يســير سوى الرحم. ولكونها مربوطة برباطات مع الصلب ومن الجانبين فلا بدّ لهذه الرباطات أن تمتدّ أيضا وتتراجع مع الرحم، وتتبعها في ذهابها ومجيئها فتسلم بذلك من التقطيع ويسلم الرحم. رابعة عشرة المنافع.

٢٤. مزاج العصب أبرد من مزاج غيره ولذلك صار البرد يؤثّر فيه سريعا ويوصل ما يناله منه إلى الدماغ. فلا ينبغي أن يقرب موضع العصب ولا يلقاه شــيء بارد ولا سيّما في خراجات. سادسة الحيلة.

٢٥. شــرّ المدن هي التي تكون مســتورة عن الرياح الشرقية وتهبّ فيها الرياح الحارّة والباردة. في شرحه للأولى من كتاب الأهوية.

٢٦. ســوء المزاج يضرّ بالقوى في جوهرها الخاصّ بها. وإذا كان ســوء المزاج مفرطا فهو يذهب بالقوة أيّ قوة كانت. سادسة العلل والأعراض.

٢٧. ســوء المــزاج المختلــف قــد يكــون فــي البدن كلّــه كالاستســقاء اللحمــي وفــي الحمّيــات كلّهــا ما خــلا حمّــى الدقّ. وقــد يكون فــي عضو

---

١ النفــس] التّنفــس SELBP | به] om. SGLBP || ٢ تضطــرّه] تضرّه SEL || ٥ ومن الجانبــين] ومــع الجنبين E || ٩ خراجات] الجراحات SEB || ١٠–١١ شــرّ المدن . . . الحارّة والباردة] قال بقراط إنّ كلّ مدينة موضوعة ســمت المغرب هي في كنّ من الرياح الشــرقيّة وتهبّ إليها الريــاح الحارّة والبــاردة من ناحية الفرقدين فتكــون هذه المدينة رديئة كثيرة الأمــراض اضطرارا. قال جالينوس إنّ بقراط لمّا ذكر هذه المدينة ومواضعها دلّنا بقوله إنّها أشرّ المدن كلّها لاختلاف هوائها . . . Galen, *In Hipp. De aere* 1.10.1.03809–03813 || ١٣ يذهــب بالقــوّة] بهذه القوة GS : يهدّ القوة BP

a swelling of the flesh[52]—that is, a phlegmatic swelling or a hot swelling. Any swelling of this type contains a varying bad temperament. *De inaequali intemperie.*[53]

(28) Insomnia is of two types—namely, the one in which a human being is involved in some activity with no obvious harm done to his strength, and the one which occurs without any external cause but which diminishes his strength,[54] appetite, digestion, and the other natural activities. *In Hippocratis Epidemiarum* 6.4.[55]

(29) Any very bad temperament which occurs in the heart in whatever way, be it primary or due to another internal organ, exhausts the animal faculty[56] and annuls it. In the same way, a very bad temperament of the brain is followed by weakness of the psychical faculty. This faculty is strangulated[57] when the ventricles of the brain are filled [with superfluities] and when the passages opening into those ventricles are obstructed. *De pulsu* 16.[58]

(30) The question of the strength [of the body] is a very grave one and the most important about which to be concerned. The permanence and continuance of the substance of this strength depends on a combination of three things: the substance of the pneuma, the substance of the main organs,[59] and the substance of the flesh. Each one of these is preserved by that which is congenial to it. The pneuma is preserved by the respiration of the chest and by the perspiration through all the pores of the body when it proceeds according to its nature, and also through the vapor which arises in the body[60] when it is in proper condition. The substance of the main organs[61] is preserved by solid and strong food. The flesh is preserved by food intermediate between moist and solid. *De methodo medendi* 11.[62]

(31) A good transformation of blood is the nourishment of the parts of the body through it, but a bad transformation means that it putrefies with a stinking putrefaction. A transformation of blood intermediate between good and bad means that it will turn into pus, for pus is formed from a combination of unnatural and innate heat. *In Hippocratis Aphorismos commentarius* 2.[63]

واحـد كالتربّـل وهـو ورم بلغمـي أو فـي الـورم الحـارّ. فـإنّ كلّ ورم من هذا الجنس فيه سـوء مـزاج مختلف. فـي مقالتـه في سـوء المـزاج المختلف.

٢٨. السهر ضربان فالذي يكون من اشتغال الإنسان بشيء من الأعمال لا ينال القـوة منه ضرر بيّن والذي يحدث من غير سـبب من خارج يضعف القوة ويضعف الشهوة والاستمراء وسائر الأفعال الطبيعية. في الرابعة من شرحه لسادسة ابيديميا.

٢٩. كلّ سـوء مـزاج عظيم يحدث في القلب علـى أيّ وجه كان حدوثه إمّا حدوثا أوّليا أو بسـبب عضو آخر من الأحشاء فهو ينهك القوة الحيوانية ويسقطها. وعلى هذا المثال يتبع سـوء مزاج الدماغ العظيم ضعف القوة النفسانية. أمّا اختناقها فتابـع لامتـلاء بطون الدماغ وللسـدد الكائنة في الطرق النافذة إلـى تلك البطون. سادسة عشر النبض.

٣٠. أمر القوة أمر خطر جدّا وهو أجلّ ما يعتنى به. وثبات جوهر القوة وقوامه باجتماع ثلاثة أشـياء وهي جوهر الروح وجوهر الأعضاء الأصلية وجوهر اللحم. ويحرز كلّ واحد منها بما يشـاكله. أمّا الروح فبالتنفّس الذي يكون بالصدر وبجملة مسامّ البدن إن كان ذلك يجري على طبعه وكذلك البخار المتولّد في البدن إن يكون جيّـدا. وأمّا جوهر الأعضاء الأصلية فتحفظ بالغـذاء الصلب القوي. وأمّا اللحم فيحفظ بالغذاء المتوسّط بين الرطب والصلب. حادية عشرة الحيلة.

٣١. تغيّر الدم الجيّد هو اغتذاء الأعضاء به وتغيّره الرديء هو أن يعفن عفنا معه نتن. وتغيّره المتوسّط بين الجيّد والرديء هو أن يصير مدّة وذلك أنّ تولّد المدّة يكون من الحرارة الخارجة عن الطبع ومن الغريزية معا. في شرح الثانية من الفصول.

---

١ كالتربّـل] كالترهـل ELB ‖ ٢ ورم] حـارّ add. S ‖ ١١ القـوة] هـو add. EL ‖ ١٣ فبالتنفّس] فبالنفس B

(32) Although every organ of the body attracts nourishment to itself, not all have the same attractive faculty. Therefore, the emaciation occurring to them in the case of lack of blood is not the same. The attractive faculty of the heart is the strongest, followed by [that of] the liver. Therefore, the heart never lacks its nourishment without the other organs [of the body] suffering from an extreme lack of blood. So, for this reason, we should not think, when the body seems to us emaciated due to prolonged illness, that the situation of the heart and liver regarding emaciation is the same as that of the other organs. *De marcore.*[64]

(33) A natural characteristic common to human beings and other living beings is that the heart is stronger than the liver in attracting what is useful to it and rejecting what is loathsome to it, and that the liver is more effective and stronger than the intestines and stomach, while the arteries are more effective and stronger than the veins. When the liver is full and stretched, while the stomach is empty and craving to attract [nutrition], the force of attraction shifts to the stomach, which then attracts [nutrition] from the liver. *De naturalibus facultatibus* 3.[65]

(34) The purified food which arrives from the stomach into the liver is boiled and cocted in the body of the liver and turned into blood. There the yellow and black bile superfluities are separated and attracted by the gallbladder and spleen. Then the blood—thin in substance—enters the large vessel that grows from the convex part of the liver and streams toward the upper and lower parts of the body. As long as the blood is in this vessel, it is mixed with a large amount of a thin watery liquid, which it needs to facilitate its passing through the many fine veins in the liver. When the blood reaches the broad vessel that is close to the right side of the heart, this superfluity [that is, the watery fluid] is separated and absorbed by the kidneys and then poured by them into the urinary bladder. *De usu partium* 4.[66]

٣٢ . وإن كان كلّ عضو من أعضاء البدن يجذب الغذاء إلى نفسه فليست هي كلّها في قوة الجذب متساوية . ولذلك صار هزالها عند نقصان الدم لا يتشابه . وقوة الجذب في القلب في غاية الشدّة وبعده الكبد . ولذلك لا يعدم القلب غذاءه أبدا دون أن يصير سائر أعضاء البدن إلى غاية نقصان الدم . فلذلك لا ينبغي لنا أن نتوهّم إذا رأينا البدن قد نحل من طول المرض به أنّ حال القلب والكبد في الهزال كحال سائر الأعضاء . في مقالته في الذبول .

٣٣ . الأمر الطبيعي العامّ في الناس وفي سائر الحيوان أنّ القلب يجتذب ما ينفعه ويدفع عنه ما ينافره أشدّ وأقوى من اجتذاب الكبد ودفعها وأنّ الكبد تفعل ذلك أشدّ وأقوى من الأمعاء والمعدة وأنّ العروق الضوارب تفعل ذلك أشدّ وأقوى من العروق الغير الضوارب . ومتى كانت الكبد ممتلئة متمدّدة وكانت المعدة خالية متشوّقة إلى الجذب انتقلت قوة الجذب إلى المعدة فتجذب من الكبد . في ثالثة القوى .

٣٤ . صفو الطعام الذي يصل من المعدة إلى الكبد يغلي وينضج في جرم الكبد ويستحيل دما . وهناك يتميّز الفضلتان الصفراء والسوداء ويجتذبهما كيس المرار والطحال . وينفذ الدم وهو رقيق القوام في العرق العظيم النابت من حدبة الكبد ويجري إلى جهتي البدن العليا والسفلى . وما دام الدم في هذا العرق فهو مختلط برطوبة كثيرة رقيقة مائية احتيج إليها ليسهل نفوذه في العروق التي في الكبد على كثرتها وضيقها . وإذا صار الدم إلى العرق الواسع القريب من الجانب الأيمن من القلب فثمّ تتميّز هذه الفضلة ويمتصّانها الكليتان ويسكبانها الى المثانة . رابعة المنافع .

---

٢ هزالها] هذا لها P || ٧ العامّ] العامي EL || ١٥ هذا العرق] هذه العروق EL || ١٦ كثيرة] حمرا EL || ١٨ ويمتصّانها] ويصببانها L : ويعمرانها B(?)

(35) The liver is nourished by thick red blood, the spleen by thin dark blood, and the lung by blood that is completely cocted, bright red, and spirituous.[67] *De usu partium* 4.[68]

(36) The intestines are coiled and surrounded by innumerable vessels. The mouths of these vessels penetrate into the inside of the intestines in order to grasp the good part of the food. The arteries which penetrate into the intestines take a small amount of food. *De usu partium* 4.[69]

(37) Both kidneys are nourished by attracting the watery part of the blood. The residue is the watery superfluity which they expel to the urinary bladder. The kidneys do not need a third vessel to bring them nutrition, as is the case with the gallbladder and urinary bladder. *De usu partium* 5.[70]

(38) There is no part of the body to which blood comes more completely cocted in arteries and veins than the breasts. This is so because that blood passes through the heart as it goes up and meets the heart again on its way down and is constantly moved by the movement of the chest and is heated during all this coming and going by its long stay [there] and by the length of the distance [it covers].[71] *De usu partium* 7.[72]

(39) The organs nourished with pure blood—namely, the organs on the right side—are warmer than the organs on the left side. So, do not be surprised that the right testicles in males are warmer than the left and that the right uterus [in females] is warmer than the left. Thus, it is not unreasonable [to say] that the parts on the right side produce males, and those on the left side, females. *De usu partium* 14.[73]

٣٥ . الكبـد يغتذي بدم أحمر غليظ والطحال يغتذي بدم لطيف أسـود والرئة تغتذي بدم قد نضج غاية النضج مشرق الحمرة قريب من طبيعة الروح. رابعة المنافع .

٣٦ . الأمعـاء كلّها تدور محوطة بعـروق لا يحصى عددها . تنفذ أفواهها إلى جوف المعاء لتخطف الشيء الجيّد من الغذاء . والعروق الضوارب النافذة إلى الأمعاء قد تأخذ من الغذاء جزءا يسيرا . رابعة المنافع .

٣٧ . الكليتـان تغتذي بما تجذب مـن مائية الدم. والبقية هي الفضلة المائية التي تدفعها للمثانة. واستغنتا الكليتان عن عرق ثالث يأتيهما يغذوهما كما يجيء لكيس المرارة والمثانة. خامسة المنافع .

٣٨ . ليـس في البـدن عضو يصل إليه دم قد اسـتحكم نضجـه في العروق الضوارب وغير الضوارب أكثر من اسـتحكام الدم الذي يصل إلى الثديين. وذلك أنّ هذا الدم يمرّ بالقلب في صعوده ويلقاه أيضا في انحداره ويتحرّك دائما بحركة الصدر ويسخن بطول تردّده لطول مكثه ولبعد المسافة. سابعة المنافع .

٣٩ . الأعضاء التي تغتذي بالدم النقي وهي الأعضاء التي في الجانب الأيمن أحرّ من الأعضاء التي في الجانب الأيسـر . فليس لك أن تعجب من فضل حرارة البيضة اليمنى من الذكور والرحم اليمنى على البيضة اليسرى والرحم اليسرى . فليس بالمنكر أن تكون الأعضاء التي في الجانب الأيمن تولد ذكورا والتي في الجانب الأيسـر تولد إناثا . رابعة عشرة المنافع .

---

٣ كلّهـا] كمـا add. ELB | تـدور] om. B | محوطـة] محيطـة L || ٤ المعاء] الأمعاء ELB || ١٠ يصل] يجيء EL || ١٢ لطول] وطول L | ولبعد] لبعد EL

(40) Since the breasts and uteri were created for a single task only, they have been joined by means of arteries and veins. The origins of these joined vessels are different from those of the other vessels. [This is because] some begin above the diaphragm and descend to the lower parts [of the body], while others begin below and pass upward, so that, during pregnancy, all that is contained in these vessels goes to the uterus and afterwards, during nursing, to the breasts. *De usu partium* 14.[74]

(41) There are five movements[75] [of the stomach], and they follow each other in proper arrangement and order. The first is evacuation, the second is the natural appetite of the emptied parts, the third is the absorption of the vessels of the stomach, the fourth is the sensation of absorption experienced by the stomach [itself], and the fifth and last one is the natural desire[76] of the stomach, which is [the same as] hunger. *De [morborum] causis et symptomatibus* 4.[77]

(42) There are five functions [of the voice], which follow each other [in proper arrangement and order]. These are the exhalation of air through breathing, exsufflation[78] with [noise, exsufflation] without noise, sound, and speech. When one of these [functions] is damaged, all the following ones are damaged [as well], but not the previous ones. *De locis affectis* 4.[79]

(43) Exhalation of air through breathing is effected through the muscles of the chest. A strong exsufflation is effected by the intercostal muscles. Noiseless exsufflation[80] is effected by pharyngeal muscles. Sound is produced by the larynx and its muscles. Speech is accomplished by the tongue, with the assistance of the teeth, lips, nostrils, uvula, and upper palate.[81] *De locis affectis* 4.[82]

٤٠ . لمّا كان الثديان والأرحام إنّما خلقا لعمل واحد أشرك بينهما بعروق ضوارب وغير ضوارب . وصارت هذه العروق المشتركة مبادئها مباينة لمبادئ سائر العروق . وذلك أنّ بعضها يبتدئ من فوق الحجاب وينحدر إلى أسفل وبعضها يبتدئ من أسفل ويرتقي إلى فوق ليكون ما في تلك العروق كلّها يصير إلى الرحم في حين الحمل ثمّ يصير كلّه إلى الثديين في حال الرضاعة . أربعة عشر المنافع .

٤١ . هاهنا خمس حركات يتلو بعضها بعضا على نسق ونظام . أوّلها الاستفراغ والثاني الشهوة الطبيعية التي في الأعضاء المستفرغة والثالث امتصاص العروق للمعدة والرابع حسّ المعدة بهذا الامتصاص والخامس شهوتها النفسانية وهو آخرها وهو الجوع . رابعة العلل والأعراض .

٤٢ . هاهنا خمسة أفعال يتلو بعضها بعضا وهو خروج الهواء بالتنفّس والنفخة التي لا قرعة معها والنفخة التي معها قرعة والصوت والكلام . ومتى نالت الفعل الواحد من هذه الخمسة مضرّة إنضرّ كلّ ما بعده ولا ينضرّ ما قبله . رابعة التعرّف .

٤٣ . إخراج الهواء بالتنفّس يفعله عضل الصدر . والنفخة القوية يفعلها العضل التي فيما بين الأضلاع . والنفخة التي لا قرعة معها يفعلها عضل الحلق . والصوت يفعله الحنجرة وعضلها . والكلام يتمّ باللسان وتعينه الأسنان والشفتان وثقبي المنخرين وأعالي اللهاة والحنك . رابعة التعرّف .

---

٦ بعضا] لبعض B || ١٠ يتلو] يتبع Galen, *De loc. aff.* 107a | وهو] وهي Galen, *ibid.* || ١٢ الواحد] الأوّل Galen, *ibid.* | الخمسة] الأفعال التي ذكرناها Galen, *ibid.* | إنضرّ . . . قبله] أضرّ ذلك بجميع الأربعة الأفعال الآخر Galen, *ibid.* || ١٣ عضل الصدر] العضل الذي يقبض الصدر Galen, *De loc. aff.* 107b | القوية] الشديدة add. Galen, *ibid.* | يفعلها] خاصّة add. Galen, *ibid.* || ١٤ لا] om. Galen, *ibid.* | والصوت] وأمّا الصوت Galen, *ibid.* || ١٥ الحنجرة وعضلها] عضل الحنجرة Galen, *ibid.* || ١٦ وأعالي اللهاة والحنك] ولأعلى الحنك واللهاة Galen, *De loc. aff.*, 108a : وأعلى الحنك واللهاة E | والحنك] في ذلك معونة add. L and Galen, *ibid.*

(44) That which nature cannot turn[83] into food as part of its transformation activity is that which settles in the urine. It does not change and turn into blood,[84] and it is not like pus, which is generated by [nature] in normal and abnormal circumstances.[85] *In Hippocratis Prognostica commentarius* 1.[86]

(45) Says Moses: What is evident to me—and this is a necessary logical conclusion—is that the food which nature cannot turn into blood in the liver is the crude chyme that appears in some urines.[87] And that which nature cannot transform into blood reaching the organs and feeding them is the sediment which appears in the urine of ill people and of some healthy people.

(46) Not only does the nutrition of the organs come from the blood, but also the protection of the innate heat. Therefore, when the quantity of blood changes because it is greatly increased or diminished, or when the quality of blood changes because it becomes very hot or it loses much of its heat, the innate heat is corrupted.[88] When this happens in the heart, its corruption extends to the whole body. When it happens in an organ far from the heart, that corruption affects the heat of that organ only, unless it extends so much beyond that organ that it reaches the heart. *De [curandi ratione per] venae sectionem.*[89]

(47) The veins that reach the brain expel the superfluities they contain into the ventricles of the brain, but retain and keep the blood they contain. *De usu partium* 9.[90]

(48) It is a natural condition that the skin is not stretched[91] while there is an empty space between the skin and the flesh. Similarly, the spaces[92] in the flesh itself are all empty, especially those around the arteries [to accommodate] their expansion.[93] In the case of hot tumors, all these spaces fill and the skin is stretched. When the tumor is chronic, pus extends to the tunics, membranes, and vessels, down to the bone below the tumor.

٤٤ . الشــيء الذي يفوت الطبيعة أن تعمل فيه من الغذاء عند إحالته هو الذي يرســب في البول . فلا يســتحيل ويصيــر دما ولا هو بمنزلة المدّة التــي تفعلها الحال الطبيعية والحال الخارجة عن الطبع . في شرحه للأولى من تقدمة المعرفة .

٤٥ . قال موســى : الذي يبدو إليّ وهو الذي يقتضيه القياس هو أنّ الذي يفوت الطبيعــة مــن الغذاء أن تحيله دما في الكبد هو الخام الــذي يظهر في بعض الأبوال . والــذي يفوت الطبيعة من إحالة الــدم الواصل إلى الأعضاء عن تغذية تلك الأعضاء هو الرسوب الذي يظهر في أبوال المرضى وبعض الأصحّاء .

٤٦ . الــدم ليــس إنّما يكون عنه اغتــذاء الأعضاء فقط بل وحراســة الحرارة الغريزيــة . فلذلك متى تغيّرت كمّية الدم بأن تكثر جدّا أو تقلّ جدّا أو تغيّرت كيفيته بأن تسخن جدّا أو تنقص حرارته نقصانا كثيرا فسدت الحرارة الغريزية . إن كان ذلك في القلب عمّ فســادها الجســم كلّه . وإن كان في عضو بعيد عن القلب كان ذلك الفساد في حرارة ذلك العضو فقط إلا أن يتعدّى من العضو إلى أن يصل إلى القلب . في مقالته في الفصد .

٤٧ العــروق الغير ضوارب التي تأتي الدماغ تقذف ما فيها من الفضل إلى بطون الدماغ وتحتبس بما فيها من الدم وتتحفّظ به . في تاسعة المنافع .

٤٨ . الحال الطبيعية أن يكون الجلد غير متمدّد وبين اللحم والجلد خال . وكذلك مواضع في نفس اللحم خالية كلّها وبخاصّة المواضع التي حول الشريانات لانبساطها فيها . فأمّا في الأورام الحارّة فتمتلئ هذه المواضع كلّها ويتمدّد الجلد . وإذا أزمن الورم يسري من المادّة للأغشية والصفاقات والعروق حتى العظم التي تحت الورم . وبالجملة

---

٢ تفعلها] تفعل SGBP || ٤ إليّ] لي LBP || ١٢ فسادها] فساده EL

In general, there is no organ that remains in the same natural condition if it is affected by a hot tumor that has become chronic. *De tumoribus [praeter naturam].*[94]

(49) There are two types of heat in the body. One is innate, and its substance lies in the blood; and the other is biting while it burns. Under this [last] category [of heat] falls fever; and this [heat] is called "strange heat," "unnatural heat," and also "acquired heat." *In Hippocratis Epidemiarum* 6.4.[95]

(50) The vessels through which food is transported from the stomach to all the organs are precisely the ones through which many superfluities stream from all the organs to the stomach and intestines in a time of purgation through drugs and in times of crises [of diseases]. In the case of healthy people, it often happens in a time of severe hunger that pure blood streams to the stomach in order to feed it. Sometimes the phlegm originating in the stomach ascends to the liver, together with the food that ascends to it. *De atra bile.*[96]

(51) Wind sometimes collects beneath the skin, and sometimes beneath the membranes covering the bones or beneath the membrane covering one of the internal organs.[97] *De methodo medendi,* last treatise.[98]

(52) The crystalline, vitreous, and albuminoid humors, and likewise the hornlike tunic, do not contain any vessels at all. The crystalline humor is nourished from the vitreous humor by transudation,[99] and the vitreous [humor] is nourished from what reaches it from the netlike tunic, which has many arteries and veins. Similarly, the hornlike [tunic] is nourished by transudation from what reaches it from the grapelike tunic, for the grapelike [tunic] also has many vessels. *De usu partium* 10.[100]

From the exits of the nerves, arteries and veins enter the spine in order to carry out the same task as with the other parts. *De usu partium* 13.[101]

Soft nerves were joined to the parts that require minute sensation and hard nerves to the parts that require voluntary motion. Hard and soft nerves

فليس من الأعضاء عضو يبقى على حاله الطبيعية في العضو الحادث فيه الورم الحارّ إذا أزمن. في مقالته في الأورام.

٤٩. في البدن حرارتان أحداهما الغريزية وجوهرها في الدم والأخرى حرّيفة تلذع. وتدخل في هذا الجنس الحمّى وهذه تسمّى حرارة غريبة وتسمّى خارجة عن الطبيعة وتسمّى أيضا حرارة مكتسبة. في الرابعة من شرحه السادسة ابيديميا.

٥٠. العروق التي فيها ينبعث الغذاء من البطن إلى جميع الأعضاء فيها بأعيانها تنصبّ فضول كثيرة من جميع الأعضاء إلى البطن والأمعاء في وقت إسهال الأدوية ووقت البحرانات. وكثيرا ما يعرض للأصحّاء في وقت الجوع الشديد أن ينصبّ إلى المعدة دم خالص ليغذوها. والبلغم الذي يتولّد في المعدة قد يرتفع إلى الكبد مع ما يرتفع إليها من الأغذية. في مقالته في المرّة السوداء.

٥١. الريح مرّة يكون اجتماعها تحت الجلد ومرّة تحت الأغشية المغشّية للعظام أو المغشّية للعضل أو تحت الغشاء المغشّي لواحد من الأعضاء الباطنة. آخر الحيلة.

٥٢. الرطوبة الجليدية والزجاجية والبيضية وكذلك الطبقة القرنية لا عروق فيها بوجه. وإنّما تغتذي الرطوبة الجليدية برشح الرطوبة الزجاجية والزجاجية بما يصلها من الطبقة الشبكية التي هي كثيرة العروق الضوارب وغير الضوارب. وكذلك القرنية تغتذي بما يرشح لها من الطبقة العنبية لأنّ العنبية أيضا كثيرة العروق. عاشرة المنافع.

يدخل إلى النخاع من مخارج العصب عروق ضاربة وغير ضاربة لتقوم لها بما تقوم لسائر الأعضاء. ثالثة عشرة المنافع.

الأعضاء التي تحتاج لحسّ لطيف وصل بها عصب ليّن والأعضاء المحتاجة إلى الحركة الإرادية وصل بها عصب صلب ووصل بالأعضاء التي تحتاج إلى الأمرين

---

١٢ آخر] أخير ELP || ١٧ بما تقوم لسائر] مقام سائرE

were joined to the parts needing both things.[102] Many nerves or large nerves have been joined to the part that needs much sensation, while no nerve has been joined to a part that does not need sensation.[103] *De usu partium* 16.

No separate, special nerve was made to reach the skin, but it is reached by certain fine subdivisions of the nerves from the parts that lie beneath it. [These subdivisions] go to these parts in order to serve as bonds between the skin and the parts beneath it and to serve as sensory organs for them. *De usu partium* 16.[104]

(53) Just as the skin has sensation[105]—although no special nerves reach it, since it receives only the faculty of sensation from the nerves, but not the faculty of motion, [with the result] that it does not move—so, too, the membranes, tunics, arteries, veins, uteri, intestines, urinary bladder,

جميعا عصب صلب وعصب ليّن. والعضو المحتاج لحسّ كثير وصل به عصب كثير أو كبير وما لا يحتاج ألى حسّ لم يوصل به عصب. سادسة عشرة المنافع.

لم يجعل للجلد عصبة تأتيه مفردة له خاصّة وإنّما تأتيه من الأعضاء المستبطنة له أقسام دقاق من أقسام العصب التي يأتي تلك الأعضاء ليكون رباطا للجلد بما يستبطنه من الأعضاء ليقوم له مقام آلة يحسّ بها. سادسة عشرة المنافع.

٥٣. كما يعمّ الحسّ للجلد فإنّ ما يأتيه عصب يخصّه لأنّه استفاد من العصب قوة الحسّ فقط لا قوة الحركة ولا يتحرّك كذلك تحسّ أيضا ولا تتحرّك الأغشية والصفاقات والعروق الضوارب وغير الضوارب والأرحام والأمعاء والمثانة والمعدة

---

٢ أو كبير] om. SB | المنافع] قد كنت علمت بالتشريح أنّ كلّ واحدة من العصب نراها عند مخرجها منشأها ملتأمة في نفسها مفردة عن غيرها بمنزلة العرق حتى يظنّ أنّها عصبة واحدة كما أنّ العرق واحد وأنّ كلّ واحدة من هذه العصب منذ أوّل أمرها ومبدأ منشئها هي عصابات كثيرة مشدودة موثوقة كلّها بلفائف تشملها وهذه اللفائف من ذينك الغشائش الملفوفين على النخاع وعلى الدماغ. في الأولى من التعرّف add. EL = Galen, *De loc. aff.* 1.6 (ed. Kühn, vol. 8, p. 57) || ٤ بما] كما SGBP || ٥ المنافع] السبب في كون بعض الأعضاء يبطل حسّه دون حركته وبعضها تبطل حركته دون حسّه على ما يظهر عيانا بيّنا لمن له علم بتشريح العصب وهو هذا أقول إنّ كلّ حركة إرادية فإنّما هي من العضل وذلك أنّه ليس من العصب واحدة تفعل في أعضاء الحيوان مثل هذا الفعل وهي مفردة بنفسها خلوا من عضلة ولا في العصب واحدة تفعل هذا ولا منه شيء يفعل ذلك في شيء من الأعضاء بل العصب كلّه يفعل ما يفعله من الحركات الإرادية بتوسّط العضل دائما وأمّا العضل فمنحدره إلى الأعضاء التي يريد أن تتحرّك مرّة يكون بلا متوسّط ومرّة يكون بمتوسّط وهي الوتر والأوتار قد يسمّيها قوم أطراف وغايات عصبانية. والأوتار المحرّكة للعصابع هي من هذا الجنس وهي مدوّرة مثل الأجزام التي يسمّيها ابقراط طريف. فمتى كانت الآفة الحادثة بعضل الأصابع فالذي يتعطّل من الأصابع حاسّة اللمس. في الأوّل من التعرّف add. EL = Galen, *De loc. aff.* 1.6 (ed. Kühn, vol. 8, pp. 59–60) || ٦ فإنّ ما] فإنّما S : فإنّ ما يأتيه وإن لم يأته LBP | يأتيه] من add. S

stomach, and all the viscera have sensation but no motion, although the nerves have both faculties, while the instrument of motion is the muscle. *De usu partium* 16.[106]

(54) One should not be amazed that, if the skin overlying a muscle loses its sensation, the movement of that muscle is not abolished; [this is] because the nerve that spreads in that muscle has not been damaged, whereas that part [of the nerve] that spreads within the skin was damaged. So, if the skin is pulled from the muscle, it is impossible for that muscle to move without having sensation. But it is possible that the muscle has sensation without motion; this occurs when the muscle is so severely damaged that, [although] the amount of power it receives from the psychical faculty is still enough [to allow] sensation through being affected, [it is] not enough for motion, because motion is [a form of] activity, while sensation is [a form of] passivity. *De [morborum] causis et symptomatibus* 4.[107]

(55) Twitching occurs in all the parts that can stretch [but never occurs in bones and cartilages,][108] because bones and cartilages do not stretch in any way. Therefore, twitching occurs frequently in the skin, and sometimes it happens also in the muscles which are beneath it. It also happens in the stomach, the urinary bladder, the uterus, the intestines, the liver, the spleen, the diaphragm, the arteries, and the heart itself. *De [morborum] causis et symptomatibus* 5.[109]

(56) In soft flesh and that which is generally called flesh,[110] only the alterative faculty is similar to that in other organs. The remaining three faculties are weaker in the flesh than in the other organs. Therefore, the soft flesh is quicker to receive [superfluous] matters than the other organs. Second—after the soft flesh—in rapidity of reception of the [superfluous] matters comes the lung, because of the softness of its substance and because of the weakness of the other three faculties in it. After the lung in rapidity of reception of the [superfluous] matters comes the spleen. The brain is similar to the spleen in rapidity of reception of the [superfluous]

وجميع الأحشـــاء وإن كان في العصـــب القوتان جميعا وآلـــة الحركة هي العضلة. سادسة عشرة المنافع.

٥٤. ليس من العجب أن يكون الجلد الذي على العضلة يتعطّل حسّه ولا يتعطّل حركـــة العضلـــة لأنّ العصبة التي تنبثّ وتتفرّق في العضلـــة لا مضرّة فيها وما يتفرّق وينبـــثّ منها في الجلد نالته مضرّة. فأمّا إن كشـــط الجلد عـــن العضلة فلا يمكن أن تتحـــرّك تلك العضلة ولا تحسّ. لكـــن من الممكن أن تحسّ ولا تتحرّك وذلك أنّ تلك العضلـــة عرضت لها مضرّة عظيمة حتى صارت إنّما تقبل من القوة النفســـانية قدرا يفـــي بأن تحسّ بالانفعال ولا تقـــدر أن تتحرّك إذ التحريك فعل والحسّ انفعال. رابعة العلل والأعراض.

٥٥. الاختـــلاج يعرض فـــي جميع الأعضاء التي يمكن أن تنبســـط لأنّ العظام والغضاريف لا تنبســـط أصلا. ولذلك يكثر الاختـــلاج في الجلد وربّما حدث أيضا في العضل الذي تحته. ويعرض في المعدة والمثانة والأرحام والأمعاء والكبد والطحال والحجاب وفي العروق الضوارب وفي القلب نفسه. خامسة العلل والأعراض.

٥٦. اللحـــم الرخو وما يســـمّى لحما على الإطلاق القـــوة المغيّرة فيه فقط مثلها في ســـائر الأعضاء. وأمّا الثلاث قوى الباقية فهي في اللحم أضعف منها في ســـائر الأعضاء. ولذلك يســـرع إليه قبول الموادّ أكثر من سائر الأعضاء. والثاني بعد اللحم الرخو في ســـرعة قبول الموادّ الرئة لرخاوة جرمها ولضعف القوى الثلاث فيها. وبعد الرئة في سرعة قبول الموادّ الطحال. وأمّا الدماغ فشبيه بهذه في سرعة قبول الموادّ أو

---

١ وإن . . . العضلة] om. B ‖ ٥ كشـــط] قشـــط ELBP ‖ ١٠ يعرض] يحدث EL ‖ ١١ ولذلك] كذلك G | حدث أيضا] عرض أيضا وحدث EL ‖ ١٧ الرئة] إليه S

matters or even more so, but it is superior to it in the quality of its composition—namely, the spaciousness of its ventricles, the large quantity of passages for its superfluities, and the fact that these passages run from top to bottom. *De [curandi ratione per] venae sectionem.*[111]

(57) Every strong organ sends its strength to a weaker organ that is near to it. Thus, the weaker organ attains a strength that is comprised of its own specific power and of the power sent to it. *In Hippocratis De alimento commentarius* 1.[112]

(58) Sometimes the body is at rest and ease when its temperament is bad because of sharp, bad humors. If the rest and ease last for a long time, this causes fever. Sometimes the rest dries the body, because it weakens the organs so that they are not well nourished. And when the body is not [well] nourished, it becomes dry and arid. *De somno et vigilia.*[113]

(59) The matters that develop in all the tumors and humors that form in arteries and veins when there is an obstruction are all of one and the same order. For, when the alterative and ripening faculty in those organs which have a tumor or in those vessels that have a humor becomes stable and strong, it transforms that which is within the tumors into good white pus, balanced in its consistency, and transforms that which is in the vessels into the sediment which settles in the urine. This kind of putrefaction is not merely putrefaction but is mixed with coction. But when the alterative faculty is very weak, there is an absolute putrefaction; and those various fluids are exuded from the tumors and those bad sediments settle in the urine of those suffering from fever. *De [differentiis] febribum* 1.[114]

(60) Nature often purges the whole body in [the case of] illness, in the [case] of the ingestion of a purgative or emetic, and in the case of cholera, while the superfluities come and go through the very same vessels by which the organs are nourished. Thus, the superfluities pass from one

أكثر إلا أنّه يفضل عليها بجودة تركيبه وهي سعة بطونه وكثرة مجاري فضوله وكونها تندفع من فوق إلى أسفل. في مقالته في الفصد.

٥٧. كلّ عضو قوي يبعث قوته إلى ما يليه من الأعضاء الضعيفة. فيحصل في الضعيف قوة مركبة من قوته الخاصّية به ومن القوة المنبعثة إليه. في شرحه لأولى الغذاء.

٥٨. ربّما سكن البدن السكون والدعة إذا كان البدن رديء المزاج فيه أخلاط حرّيفة رديئة. وإن طال السكون والدعة عرض من ذلك حمّى. وربّما يبّس السكون البدن بإضعافه الأعضاء فلا تغتذي غذاء جيّدا. وإذا لم يغتذِ البدن يبس وجفّ. في مقالته في النوم واليقظة.

٥٩. الموادّ التي تكون في جميع الأورام والأخلاط التي تكون في العروق الضوارب وغير الضوارب إذا كانت هناك سدد حال الجميع حال واحدة. وذلك أنّ القوة المغيّرة المنضجة التي في تلك الأعضاء التي فيها الورم أو في تلك العروق التي فيها الخلط إن كانت ثابتة قوية أحالت ما في الأورام إلى مدّة جيّدة بيضاء معتدلة القوام وأحالت ما في العروق الى الثفل الذي يرسب في البول. وهذا الجنس من العفونة ليس هو عفونة فقط بل يشوبه نضج. وإن كانت تلك القوة المغيّرة قد ضعفت جدّا كان العفن المطلق وخرج من الأورام تلك الرطوبات المختلفة ورسب في البول من المحمومين تلك الأثفال المذمومة. في الأولى من الحمّيات.

٦٠. كثيرا ما تنقّي الطبيعة جميع البدن في الأمراض وفي وقت تناول الدواء المسهل والمقيّئ وفي حال الهيضة ويكون مجيء الفضول وخروجها في تلك العروق بأعيانها التي منها اغتذت الأعضاء. حتى تجيء تلك الفضول من عضو إلى عضو

١ أكثر] أفضل B | بطونه] برطوبته B || ٤ الخاصّية به] الكائنة فيه L || ٥ سكن] سخن SGP || ١٢ ثابتة] تابعة (!)B || ١٧ كثيرا] om. B

organ to another until they reach the vessels spreading from the intestines and stomach. No wonder, then, that nutriment returns from the outer skin surface to the depths of the body, and that it reaches the stomach [as it returns] from the liver and spleen through the very same vessels through which it ascended from the stomach [initially]. *De naturalibus facultatibus* 3.[115]

(61) If fluids stream into the cavities of organs that have tumors and remain there for a long time, they undergo a great variety of transformations. In the case of abscesses, one often finds substances similar to stones, sand, potsherds, wood, coal, sediment of olive oil, lees of wine, and other substances of different sorts. *Ad Glauconem [de methodo medendi]* 2.[116]

(62) The penis, genitalia, and neck of the uterus are reached by a surplus of nerves because of the extra sensation which they need during sexual intercourse. The other procreative parts, such as the uteri as a whole [and] the male testicles with their receptacle—that is, the scrotum—are reached [only] by small nerves like the nerves which reach the other internal parts, such as the liver, spleen, and kidneys. *De usu partium* 14.[117]

(63) When blood streams to empty places and a tumor forms [in an organ], if the innate heat of that organ has greatly deviated from its equilibrium, that blood putrefies just as the bodies of the dead do.[118] But, if the innate heat remains [in a balanced state] and does not deviate too much from it, it prevails over that blood and transforms it into pus. According to the variation in these two circumstances, the conditions of the pus vary in proximity to putrefaction or to coction. *In Hippocratis Prognostica commentarius* 1.[119]

(64) When the vessels of any muscle fill with [so much] warm blood [that] they become obstructed by it, and when their orifices open and that blood streams to those openings that are in the flesh of the muscle and those that are outside the muscle, and when the substance of the flesh of the muscle becomes hot due to what is inside it and due to what is outside it,

إلـى العروق التي تمتدّ من الأمعاء والمعدة. وليس مـن العجب أن يتراجع الغذاء من سـطح الجلد الظاهر ثانية إلى عمق البدن ولا أن يأتي إلى المعدة من الكبد والطحال في تلك العروق بأعيانها التي يتراقى فيها من المعدة. في ثالثة القوى.

٦١. إذا طـال لبـث الرطوبـات المنصبّـة إلـى خلـل الأعضـاء التـي قـد تورّمـت حـدث لهـا اسـتحالات مختلفة جـدّا. فقـد يوجد كثيـرا في الدبيـلات أجسـام شـبيهة بالحجـارة وبالرمل وبالأخـزاف والخشـب وبالفحم وبعكـر الزيـت وبالـدردي وبغيـر ذلـك مـن أنـواع شـتّى. ثانيـة أغلوقن.

٦٢. القضيـب والقبل وعنق الرحم يأتيها فضل عصب لاحتياجها لفضل حسّ عنـد الجماع. أمّا ما سـواها من بقية التوليد كجملة الأرحـام وخصيتي الذكور مع وعائهما وهو الصفن فإنّما يأتيهما عصب صغار مثل العصب الذي يأتي سائر الأعضاء الباطنة كالكبد والطحال والكليتين. رابعة عشرة المنافع.

٦٣. إذا اندفـع الـدم للمواضع الخاليـة وحدث الـورم إن كان ذلك العضو قد خرجـت حرارته الغريزية عـن اعتداله خروجا كثيرا عفن ذلك الدم كما تعفن أبدان الموتى. وإن كانت باقية ولم تخرج خروجا كثيرا قويت على ذلك الدم وأحالته مدّة. وبحسب اختلاف هاتين الحالتين تختلف أحوال المدّة في القرب من العفن أو النضج. في شرحه للأولى من تقدمة المعرفة.

٦٤. إذا امتـلأت العروق التي فـي عضلة من العضل دما حـارّا وغصّت به وانفتحت فوهاتها وسـال ذلك الدم لتلك الفرج التي في لحم العضلة والفرج التي من خارج العضلة وصار جوهر لحم العضلة يسـخن بما هـو داخله وبما هو خارج عنه

---

١ تورّمت] تفرقت B ‖ ٩ وخصيتي] وبيضتي B ‖ ١٧ وغصّت به] وجذبته < . . . > L : وجات به EO ‖ ١٩ بما] ممّا ELO

then the flesh will be of a varying bad temperament and cause a sensation of pain as long as it is affected in this way. When the heat prevails over the muscle as a whole and the heat of the flesh at the inside and outside is equal, the bad temperament of the muscle does not vary anymore but becomes even, and the sensation of pain stops. The same holds [true]—as you should understand—for all the [other] parts of the body. *De inaequali intemperie.*[120]

(65) Sometimes a bad humor resembling a deadly poison collects in the body and has a gradual effect on the organs of the body. When it reaches its maximum malignancy, its effects become visible all at once, and it kills rapidly. Just as the effect of deadly drugs depends on their quality and not on their quantity, in the same way one should imagine that [the effect of] diseases which cause agitation and kill rapidly is as if someone takes a deadly drug or is bitten by a viper. *In Hippocratis Epidemiarum* 3.3.[121]

(66) The parts that get tired first are those that receive the defluxion descending from the head. When fatigue occurs through the voice, it results in angina; when it occurs through the hand, paralysis[122] occurs; and, when it occurs through riding, pain in the back develops. The same happens with the other parts. *In Hippocratis Epidemiarum* 6.7.[123]

(67) The most important and most dangerous element in treating diseases is a bad temperament. This is so because the temperament is the most important of the kinds [of things existing] in nature. *De methodo medendi* 7.[124]

(68) The strongest cause in the generation of diseases is the predisposition of the body which is likely to fall ill.[125] Therefore, not all people die during the course of an epidemic, nor do all of them fall ill with the rise of Sirius. *De [differentiis] febribum* 1.[126]

(69) An extreme change in weather[127] causing illness, overeating to the point of oppressing one's strength, excessive physical exercise, excessive bathing, and excessive sleep are all counted among the unnatural

فطال ما اللحم في هذا الانفعال فهو في سوء مزاج مختلف ويحسّ به الألم. فإذا استحوذت الحرارة على العضلة كلّها وكانت سخونة اللحم باطنه وظاهره شيئًا واحدا فقد ارتفع الاختلاف وصار حينئذ للعضلة سوء مزاج مستو ويرتفع الإحساس بالألم. وهكذا فافهم في الأعضاء كلّها. في مقالته في سوء المزاج المختلف.

٦٥. قد يجتمع في البدن خلط رديء شبيه بالسمّ القاتل ويعمل قليلا قليلا في أعضاء البدن. وإذا بلغ إلى غاية الرداءة ظهرت أفعاله بغتة فقتل بسرعة. وكما أنّ الفاعل في الأدوية القتّالة كيفيتها لا كمّيتها كذلك ينبغي أن يتوهّم على الأمراض التي تهيج فتقتل بسرعة كما لو تناول إنسان دواء قتّالا أو نهشته أفعى. في الثالثة من شرحه من ابيديميا.

٦٦. الأعضاء التي تقدّم لها التعب هي التي تقبل النزلة المنحدرة من الرأس. فإن كان التعب بالصوت حدثت الذبحة أو باليد حدث الفالج أو بالركب حدث وجع الظهر. وكذلك في سائر الأعضاء. في سابعة من شرحه لسادسة ابيديميا.

٦٧. أجلّ ما في تدبير الأمراض قدرا وأعظمه خطرا سوء المزاج. لأنّ جنس المزاج أجلّ ما في الطبع قدرا. سابعة الحيلة.

٦٨. أقوى الأسباب في توليد الأمراض إنّما هو استعداد البدن القابل للآفة. ولذلك لا يموت الناس كلّهم عند حدوث الموتان ولا يمرضون كلّهم عند طلوع الشعرى العبور. في الأولى من الحمّيات.

٦٩. تغاير الهواء المفرطة الممرّضة وكثرة الطعام حتى يثقل القوة وإفراط الرياضة وكذلك إفراط الاستحمام وإفراط النوم كلّ هذه تعدّ من الأسباب الخارجة عن الطبيعة

---

٧ القتّالة] القاتلة SB | كيفيتها] بكيفيتها GB || ١٠ بالركب] بالركوب ELBOP || ١٢ تدبير] تركيب B(!)

causes, for an excess in these natural [causes] makes them unnatural—they become unnatural, although they are a kind [of cause] which is not unnatural [by itself]. *De pulsibus libellus [ad tirones].*[128]

(70) Weak powers often decline and suffer defeat from minor causes, while strong powers are overcome and subdued only by major causes. Therefore, strong bodies that remain free from diseases for a long time come within sight of ruin when they fall ill. But weak bodies which constantly fight afflictions escape from diseases and are saved from them in the easiest of ways. *De pulsu* 14.[129]

(71) If someone enjoys lasting and constant health, strong causes will not alter his body. But, in the case of old men, convalescents, and all sickly people, the slightest cause produces a great change in their bodies. Similarly, if an old man or convalescent only slightly exceeds the proper bounds in the quantity or quality of food, [he] suffers great harm therefrom. But young people suffer only slight harm from serious offenses [against their health]. *De sanitate tuenda* 5.[130]

(72) Intrinsically, corruption occurs to a living being, first of all, in two ways: either through [the being's] drying up and growing old, which results in death, or through the constant dissolution of his essence—namely, the innate heat—which also results in death. But corruption also occurs to a living being in another way intrinsically connected to the food and drink he consumes—[that is,] through the production of superfluities in him. All these things [occur] intrinsically. But corruption also occurs to him through extrinsic [means]: one of them is inseparable (namely, the air), and the other is occasional (namely, the other things which change his temperament). *De sanitate tuenda* 1.[131]

(73) [In the case of] one whom you find who falls ill only on rare occasions, do not change any of his habits in his entire regimen. But [in the case of] one who falls ill frequently, you should look for the cause of

لأنّ تزيّد هذه الأسباب التي ليست بطبيعية تخرجها لأن تصير خارجة عن الطبيعة وإن كان جنسها غير خارج عن الطبيعة. في النبض الصغير.

٧٠. القوى الضعيفة تخور وتهزم مرارا شتّى من أسباب يسيرة والقوى القوية ليس يقهرها ولا يغلبها إلا الأسباب العظيمة. ولذلك صارت الأبدان القوية التي تمكث دهرا طويلا سليمة من الأمراض إذا هي مرضت بلغت لمشارفة الهلاك. والأبدان الضعيفة التي تقارع الآفات المتوالية تنجو من المرض وتفلت منه بأسهل الوجوه. رابعة عشرة النبض.

٧١. من كانت صحته ثابتة متمكّنة فالأسباب القوية لا تغيّر بدنه. أمّا الشيوخ والناقهون وكلّ مسقام فأنّ الأسباب التي في غاية الضعف تغيّر أبدانهم تغيّرا عظيما. وكذلك إن تجاوز الشيخ والناقه في كمّية الطعام أو كيفيته تجاوزا يسيرا ناله من ذلك ضرر عظيم. أمّا الشباب فالذي ينالهم من الجنايات العظيمة يسيرا. خامسة تدبير الصحة.

٧٢. الفساد يعرض للحيوان أوّلا من ذاته على ضربين إمّا بأن يجفّ فيهرم فيصير إلى الموت وإمّا بأن يتحلّل جوهره وهو الحارّ الغريزي تحلّلا دائما فيصير أيضا إلى الفناء. ثمّ يعرض له الفساد أيضا على وجه آخر لازم لما يتناوله من الطعام والشراب بما يتولّد فيه من الفضول فهذه كلّها من ذاته. ويعرض له أيضا الفساد بأشياء خارجة عن ذاته أحدهما غير مفارق له وهو الهواء والآخر سائر ما يلقاه ممّا يغيّر مزاجه أو يفرق اتّصاله. في الأولى من تدبير الصحة.

٧٣. كلّ من وجدته لا يكاد يمرض إلا في الندرة فلا تنقله عن شيء من عاداته في جميع تدبيره. وكلّ من كان يمرض أمراضا متواترة فينبغي لك أن تبحث عن

---

٣ وتهزم] وتهرم P || ٤ تمكث] مكثت B || ٨ فالأسباب] فلو الأسباب BOP || ٩ والناقهون] من المرض add. BELP | وكلّ مسقام] والمساقم LB || ١٥ مفارق] موافق B

[the illness] and eliminate it. There is no doubt that this [should be achieved] through a change in one or more of his habits. Consider, also, [in the case of] someone whose habit you want to change, whether or not such a change can be well tolerated by him. *De sanitate tuenda* 6.[132]

(74) [In the case of] one who suffers from one illness after another because of an affliction in his body, the cause of his illness can be one of two things: either overfilling (in which case he should diminish the intake [of food and drink] into his body) or a bad humor originating in the body (in [which] case he should avoid things that produce bad humors). One should take care that one's stools are soft in either case. *De sanitate tuenda* 6.[133]

(75) The body that has become weak because of a chronic illness, evacuation, or bad humor needs moist, quickly digestible food with a fragrant, pleasant aroma. For a pleasant aroma adds [something][134] to the body, balances its bad temperament, and strengthens the innate heat. *In Hippocratis De alimento commentarius* 4.[135]

(76) Concerning chronic illnesses such as orthopnea, stones, tumors[136] in the nose, bad ulcers, and the like, most of these afflictions occurring to youngsters and children are cured in forty days or seven months or seven years. Some of them [are cured] before the pubic hair starts to grow and, in the case of girls, at the time of menstruation. *De signis mortis.*[137]

(77) When the temporal muscles suffer a blow or are harmed [in any other way], they bring on spasms, fevers, stupor, and delirium[138] more than any of the other muscles because of their proximity to the origin of the nerves. For this reason, this muscle is well protected and buried between two bones. *De usu partium* 11.[139]

(78) If the grapelike tunic is severely torn, the albuminoid humor flows out of the grapelike tunic and meets the hornlike tunic, and this results in two afflictions. One of these is that the grapelike tunic falls on

السـبب في ذلك وترفعه. ولا شـكّ أنّ ذلك بتغيير عادة من عاداته أو أكثر. وانظر أيضـا في من تنقله من عادة إلى عادة هل يحسـن احتماله لهـا أو لا يحتمل ذلك. سادسة تدبير الصحة.

٧٤. كلّ من يمرض أمراضا مترادفة لآفة في بدنه فسبب مرضهم أحد أمرين إمّا فضل امتلاء فقلّل ما يرد إلى البدن وإمّا خلط رديء يتولّد في البدن فامنع من الأشياء المولّدة له. ولا تغفل لين الطبع في كلّ نازلة. سادسة تدبير الصحة.

٧٥. البدن الذي قد ضعف لمرض مزمن أو لاستفراغ أو لخلط رديء يحتاج إلى غذاء رطب سـريع الانهضام له رائحة طيّبة لذيـذة لأنّ الرائحة الطيّبة تزيد في البدن وتعدّل مزاجه الرديء وتقوي الحرارة الغريزية. في شرحه لرابعة الغذاء.

٧٦. الأمراض المزمنة مثل ضيق النفس والحصاة والبواسـير في الأنف والقروح الرديئة ونحوها فإنّ أكثر هذه الأوجاع التي تعرض للغلمان والأطفال يبرأ إلى أربعين يوم أو إلى سـبعة أشـهر أو إلى سبعة سنين. وبعضها إلى منتهى نبات الشعر على العانة وفي الجواري إلى وقت الطمث. في مقالته في علامات الموت.

٧٧. متى أصابت ضربة أو آفة لعضلتي الصدغين كان جلبها للتشنّج والحمّيات والسبات والوسواس أكثر من سائر العضل كلّه لقربه من مبدأ العصب. ولذلك أحتيط على هذا العضل ودفن بين عظمين. حادية عشرة المنافع.

٧٨. إذا انخرقت الطبقة العنبية خرقا فاحشـا سالت الرطوبة البيضية وتخرج خارجـا عن الطبقة العنبية وتلقى الطبقة القرنية فيعرض من ذلك آفتان: أحدهما أنّ

---

١ وترفعه] وتعرفه ELO || ٢ من] om. EL || ٤ لآفة] om. ELO || ٦ نازلة] هؤلاء B || ١٤ لعضلتي] لعصبتي L : لعضل الذي في B || ١٦ ودفن] ووضع L

the crystalline humor, and the other is that pneuma escapes from that wound. *De [morborum] causis et symptomatibus* 4.[140]

(79) Tumors in the noble organs are fatal. Tumors in the other internal organs that are not noble can be fatal because of their size, or because of the [diminished] strength [of the body], or because of an error in the treatment [prescribed by the physician]. *In Hippocratis Prognostica commentarius* 1.[141]

(80) Our bodies do not remain constantly in one condition—either quantitatively, because of dissolution, or qualitatively, because of external influences. Therefore, our bodies have been provided with the nutritive faculty to correct the corruption occurring in [terms of] quantity. For the correction of the corruption occurring in [terms of] quality, [our bodies] have been provided with two kinds of respiration: one through the movement of the chest, and the other through the movement of the pulse.[142] *In Hippocratis Epidemiarum* 6.5.[143]

(81) It is difficult to preserve [one's health][144] when the stomach is hot and cold superfluities descend to it from the head, or when the stomach is cold and hot superfluities descend to it from the head. I have tested and found that, of these two [conditions], the most difficult [to treat] is [the case of] a hot stomach to which cold, phlegmatic humors descend. But the worst case is when this is combined with a dry abdomen and difficulty in vomiting.[145] *De sanitate tuenda* 6.[146]

(82) Excruciating pains caused by dryness are hard to cure or cannot be cured at all. Mostly, this dryness is associated with a fever occurring [due to] a hot tumor in the brain.[147] *De methodo medendi* 12.[148]

(83) I do not know anyone who suffered from spasms due to a hot tumor in the brain [who] was cured, nor have I heard of such a case. But spasms due to overfilling of the nervous system, or those due to a biting humor which consumes these parts, or those due to severe cold result in something similar to a hardening of the nerves.[149] These three kinds of spasms can often be cured. *De methodo medendi* 12.[150]

الطبقـة العنبية تقع على الرطوبة الجليدية والأخـرى أنّ الروح يجري ويخرج من تلك الجراحة. رابعة العلل والأعراض.

٧٩. أورام الأعضاء الشريفة قاتلة. وأمّا أورام سائر الأعضاء الباطنة غير الشريفة فقد تقتل لعظمها أو لضعف القوة أو لخطاء يقع في التدبير. في شرحه للأولى من تقدمة المعرفة.

٨٠. أبداننـا غيـر ثابتة على حـال واحدة لا في كمّيتها مـن أجل التحلّل ولا فـي كيفيتها من أجل ما يلقاها من خارج. ولذلك جعل في أبداننا لإصلاح الفسـاد الحادث في الكمّية القوة الغاذية. وجعل لإصلاح الفسـاد الحادث في الكيفية جنسا التنفّس اللذين أحدهما بحركة الصدر والآخر بحركة النبض. في الخامسة من شرحه لسادسة ابيديميا.

٨١. يعسـر الاحتياط إذا كانت المعدة حارّة وكان ينحدر إليها من الرأس فضول بـاردة أو كانت المعدة باردة تنحدر إليهـا من الرأس فضول حارّة. وجرّبت فوجدت أصعبهما المعدة الحارّة التي تنحدر إليها أخلاط باردة بلغمية. وشرّ ما يكون ذلك مع يبس البطن وعسر القيء. سادسة تدبير الصحّة.

٨٢. الوجع المبرّح من قبل اليبس عسـر البـروء أو غير قابل للبروء. وأكثر ما يعرض هذا اليبس مع الحمّى التي تكون مع ورم حارّ في الدماغ. ثانية عشرة الحيلة.

٨٣. لا أعلم أحدا أصابه التشنّج من ورم حارّ في الدماغ برأ ولا سمعت ذلك. أمّا التشـنّج الحادث عن امتلاء الأعضاء العصبانيـة أو من قبل خلط لذّاع يأكلها أو من قبل برودة قوية يحدث عنها شبيه بالجمود في الأعصاب فهذه الثلاثة أصناف من التشنّج كثيرا ما تقبل العلاج. ثانية عشرة الحيلة.

---

٣ وأمّا] وإنّما B || ٧ الكمّية . . . الحادث في] om. B || ٨ بحركة] om. LO

(84) A severe headache occurs from heat or cold. The headache occurring because of dryness is mild. Moisture is not accompanied by pain at all. A large quantity of humors in the head causes heaviness but no headache unless obstructions occur from it, because the headache is commensurate with the degree of obstruction. *Mayāmir* 2.[151]

(85) In most cases, one should not use curbing and restraining drugs for abscesses occurring in the roots of the ears[152] in the beginning of their appearance, as with other tumors. Rather, we should do the opposite—namely, treat them with attractive drugs. If this does not work, we should apply cupping glasses until the malignant, harmful humor is extracted from the inside of the body to the region of the skin. I never advise application of a restraining treatment, except for a light one when there is no pain and when the body is clean. *Mayāmir* 3.[153]

(86) When abscesses occurring in the roots of the ears[154] begin to disperse by themselves, [one should] not use anything either to stimulate [this process] or to attract [the humor]. In this case, the whole matter should be left to nature. If pus collects, one should either lance the [abscesses] so that that pus can stream out of the ear or disperse and destroy them by means of drugs. *Mayāmir* 3.[155]

(87) If hot matter runs from the head to the eye, [one should] start with a general evacuation of the body through phlebotomy or through purgation of the bowels, followed by emptying of the head, especially by gargling and by attracting the matter to the opposite side by means of cupping glasses and the like. Occasionally, we split or cut the arteries close to the ears or on the temples and then treat the eye itself. *Mayāmir* 4.[156]

(88) A phlegmatic tumor hardly ever occurs in the chest and liver because the chest is too solid, strong, and firm for this kind of matter to reach it. In the case of the liver, this is true [as well] not only because it

٨٤ . الصداع الشـــديد يعرض من الحرارة والبرودة . أمّا الصداع العارض من قبل اليبوسة فهو ضعيف . وأمّا الرطوبة فليس يعرض معها وجع بتّة . وأمّا كثرة الأخلاط فـي الرأس فتحدث ثقلا لا صداعا إلا أن حدثت عنها سـدد فـإنّ الصداع يكون بحسب مقدار السدّة . ثانية الميامر .

٨٥ . الخراجات التي تحدث في أصول الأذن لا سـبيل فيها على الأمر الأكثر أن تمنـع وتردع في أوّل ظهورها كسـائر الأورام . بل نفعـل بها ضدّ ذلك وهو أن نعالجها بأدوية تجذب . فإن لم تؤثّر اسـتعملنا المحاجم حتى تجذب الخلط الرديء الموذي من داخل البدن إلى ناحية الجلد . ولا أشير بردعه أبدا إلا في النادر قد تردعه قليل ردع إذا لم يكن هناك وجع وكان البدن نقيا . ثالثة الميامر .

٨٦ . الخراجـات التي تحدث فـي أصول الأذان إذا أخذت في التحلّل من تلقاء أنفسها فلا تحرّكها بشيء ولا تجذبها . وكل الأمر كلّه حينئذ إلى الطبيعة . فإن جمعت مدّة فإمّا أن تبطّ وتسيل تلك المدّة أو تحلّلها وتفنيها بالأدوية . ثالثة الميامر .

٨٧ . إذا كانـت مادّة حارّة تتحلّب من الرأس إلى العين فتبدأ باسـتفراغ البدن عامّــة بفصد العرق أو إسـهال البطن وبعد ذلك اسـتفراغ الـرأس خاصّة بالغرغرة واجتــذاب المادّة إلى خلاف الجهة بالحجامة ونحوها . وربّما فجّرنا العروق الضوارب أو قطعناها التي تلي الأذنين أو التي على الصدغين وبعد ذلك نداوي العين نفسـها . رابعة الميامر .

٨٨ . لا يـكاد يكون فـي الصدر والكبد ورم بلغمي لأنّ الصدر أكثف وأشـدّ اسـتحصافا من أن يصل إليه مثل هذه المادّة . وأمّا الكبد فليست لكونها أكثف فقط

---

١ العـارض] الحـادث EL || ٢ معهـا] منهـا EL || ٥ الأذن] الآذان ELB || ٧ الرديء] om. ELBP || ٨ تردعه قليل] يردع بقليل ELB || ١٠ التحلّل] التحليل E || ١٤ استفراغ] استفرغ SG || ١٩ فليست] فليس EL

is very solid, but also because it changes and transforms the nature of the food.[157] For this reason, viscous phlegm and thick blood never enter the body of the diaphragm, and especially not the nervous part of it, because of its thickness. *De pulsu* 6.[158]

(89) Weakness of either liver or stomach brings those suffering from it to ruin. Therefore, it is necessary to strengthen these organs constantly.[159] When the strength of the other organs fails, it is not dangerous. When the strength of the intestines or chest fails, one is not safe from bad consequences. However, their condition is intermediate because, to the same degree that they fall short of the eminence of liver and stomach, they surpass the other parts of the body. *De methodo medendi* 11.[160]

(90) If a tumor appears in the chest or stomach or one of the parts of the neck and head, one should bind the hands and feet. If a tumor appears in the hands, one should bind the feet; and, if a tumor appears in the feet, one should bind the hands. *De methodo medendi* 13.[161]

(91) The liver and the spleen are the quickest and most susceptible of the organs to become hard if someone neglects them through taking viscous foods. Similarly, the kidneys are quickly affected by hardness. Therefore, some renal diseases cannot be cured,[162] while others are hard to cure. *De methodo medendi* 13.[163]

(92) Pay attention and be extremely careful that no hardness occurs to liver, spleen, or kidneys. Mostly, these hard conditions[164] occur to somebody who suffers from a hot tumor in one of these three organs and then takes foods that produce coarse and viscous humors. *De methodo medendi* 13.[165]

لكنّها مع ذلك تحيل الطعام وتقلّبه عن طبيعته. ولذلك لا يدخل بدن الحجاب في وقت من الأوقات لكثافته البلغم اللزج والدم الغليظ وبخاصّة الجزء العصبي منه. سادسة النبض.

٨٩. الكبد والمعدة يؤول بأصحابها ضعف كلّ واحد منهما إلى الهلاك وشيكا. فلذلك ينبغي أن تقويهما دائما. وأمّا سائر الأمعاء إن ضعفت قواها فلا خطر في ذلك. وأمّا الكليتان والصدر فضعف قوّاها ممّا لا يؤمن سوء عاقبته. لكنّ حالها حال متوسّطة لأنّها بحسب تقصيرها عن جلالة الكبد والمعدة تفوق سائر الأعضاء. حادية عشرة الحيلة.

٩٠. إذا تورّم الصدر أو المعدة أو أحد أعضاء الرقبة والرأس فشدّ اليدين والرجلين. وإن تورّمت اليدان فشدّ الرجلين وإن تورّمت الرجلان فشدّ اليدين. ثالثة عشرة الحيلة.

٩١. الكبد والطحال أسرع الأعضاء وأكثرها استعدادا لقبول الصلابة متى توانى الإنسان عنها في استعمال الأطعمة اللزجة. وكذلك الكليتان يعرض لهما الصلابة سريعا. ولذلك صار بعض علل الكليتين لا ينحلّ وبعضها يعسر انحلالها. ثالثة عشرة الحيلة.

٩٢. اجعل وكدك واحرص غاية الحرص ألا يحدث للكبد والطحال والكلى صلابة. وأكثر ما تعرض هذه الأورام الصلبة لمن يصيبه ورم حارّ في أحد هذه الثلاثة أعضاء ثمّ يستعمل أطعمة تولد أخلاطا غليظة لزجة. ثالثة عشرة الحيلة.

---

١ ولذلك] وكذلك SP || ٤ بأصحابها] بصاحبهما EL || ٩ والرأس] والرحم ELO || ١٠ ثالثة] ثانية SG || ١٣ عنها] عنهما EL || ١٦ وكدك] ذكرك B

(93) When a wound or ulcer occurs in the large intestine, it is easily healed because the large intestine is very fleshy and thick and medications settle and stay there [for a long time]. The small intestine is very difficult to heal, while the jejunum in particular cannot be healed at all when a wound occurs in it because of the thinness of its body, its extreme sensitivity,[166] its abundance of vessels, and the passing of bile through it. [The jejunum] is the only [organ] that is always free [of food]. *De methodo medendi* 6.[167]

(94) It is, above all, the outer layer of the skin[168] in which humors arriving at it are retained and become stuck—namely, those humors which are thick and earthlike. This results in mange, the disease in which the skin peels off,[169] and elephantiasis. *De medicamentis,* last treatise.[170]

(95) Marasmus develops gradually from tumors that are not dissolved or that are hidden from perception. *De pulsibus libellus [ad tirones].*[171]

(96) For the most part, the accumulation of pus[172] in hot tumors takes place after the twentieth day[173] and in cold tumors, after the sixtieth day.[174] *In Hippocratis Prognostica commentarius* 1.[175]

(97) It is in all cases unavoidable that the heart is afflicted when death occurs. Death always results from an extreme bad temperament of the heart. If the bad temperament of the heart is severe and specific for the homogeneous parts, it is not followed by a quick death. But when it is specific for the composite organs, it is followed by sudden death, which is at times preceded by severe syncope. *De locis affectis* 5.[176]

(98) It is absolutely impossible for the arteries to undergo a change affecting all of them without the heart suffering through sharing the pain with the ailing organ. The organ with which the heart shares the pain in the quickest possible way [more than the other organs] is the lung; after the lung comes the liver, and after the liver the diaphragm, and after the diaphragm the chest. *De [praesagitione ex] pulsibus* 16.[177]

٩٣ . إذا كانت الجراحة والقرحة في الأمعاء الغلاظ سهل بروءها لأنّها ألحم وأغلظ والأدوية تقف فيها وتلبث . والأمعاء الدقاق أعسر بروءا والمعاء الصائم خاصّة لا يقبل البرء بتّة إذا وقعت به جراحة لرقّة جرمه وذكاء حسّه وكثرة عروقه ومرور المرار عليه . وهو صرف بحدته دائما . سادسة الحيلة .

٩٤ . القشرة التي في ظاهر الجلد هي التي فيها خاصّة يحتبس ويلحج من الأخلاط التي تصير إلى الجلد ما هو منها غليظ أرضي . ومنه يكون الجرب والعلّة التي يتقشّر معها الجلد والجذام . آخر الأدوية .

٩٥ . قد يعرض الذبول قليلا قليلا من قبل أورام لم تنحلّ ومن قبل أورام تخفى عن الحسّ . في النبض الصغير .

٩٦ . أكثر ما يتأخّر جمع المدّة في الأورام الحارّة إلى عشرين يوما وفي الأورام الباردة إلى الستّين . في شرحه للأولى من تقدمة المعرفة .

٩٧ . لا بدّ على كلّ حال أن ينال القلب آفة عند حلول الموت . والموت إنّما هو تابع أبدا لإفراط سوء مزاج القلب . فما كان من سوء مزاج القلب عظيم المقدار وخاصّ بالأعضاء المتشابهة الأجزاء فليس يتبعه موت عاجل . وما هو منه خاصّ بالأعضاء المركّبة فالموت يتبعه فجأة ويتقدّمه الغشي القوي مرارا . خامسة التعرّف .

٩٨ . لا يمكن بتّة أن تتغيّر جميع العروق الضاربة تغيّرا يعمّها دون أن يألم القلب بمشاركته للعضو الآلم . والعضو الذي يتألّم القلب بمشاركته له في تألّمه في أسرع ما يمكن أكثر من سائر الأعضاء هو الرئة وبعد الرئة الكبد وبعد الكبد الحجاب وبعد الحجاب الصدر . سادسة عشرة النبض .

---

١ الجراحة] الخراجة B || ٣ جراحة] خراجة B || ٦ الجلد] الخلط G || ٧ والجذام] والعظام G || ١٠ المدّة] المادّة EGS

(99) If fineness of a humor, looseness [of the substance][178] of the organ, heat of the surrounding air, strength of the medicine applied, and abundant strength in the patient combine, the tumor is quickly and sometimes suddenly dissolved. But, if the opposite conditions combine, the opposite is the case. *In Hippocratis Prognostica commentarius* 2.[179]

(100) The death of ill people occurs in one of four ways: either the patient suffers an absolutely bad crisis and dies the very same day; or the strength of the patient is dissipated slowly until he dies (this is called marasmus); or both things occur together—namely, that the condition of the patient becomes very bad all of a sudden, while his strength continues to decline gradually until he dies; or, sometimes, the patient dies suddenly, without any crisis at all. *De crisibus* 3.[180]

(101) Says Moses: It is well known that this sudden death without a crisis cannot occur when the disease is abating but, rather, occurs during one of the other three stages which precede the abatement [of the disease]. Galen himself explained in his *De crisibus,* book 3, that, during the abatement of a disease, death does not occur at all unless the patient dies because of an error.[181]

(102) Any illness that subsides without a clear evacuation, or with a fairly large abscess, will return in a worse form than before. *De crisibus* 3.[182]

(103) The death of those who die without a crisis occurs on the day of the paroxysm [of the disease]. Some of them die in the beginning of fever attacks, others die when the attack reaches its peak, and yet others [die] when the attack is receding and their strength is eroded. *De crisibus* 3.[183]

(104) All the secretions[184] discharged from the body are discharged in two ways: sometimes they are discharged because the bodies which contain them remove and expel them, and sometimes they are discharged because

٩٩ . إذا اجتمع لطافة الخلط وتخلخل العضو وحرارة الهواء المحيط وقوة الدواء المستعمل وشدّة قوة المريض تحلّل الورم بسرعة وربّما تحلّل بغتة . فإذا اجتمعت أضداد هذه الأحوال كان الأمر بالضدّ . في شرحه لثانية تقدمة المعرفة .

١٠٠ . موت المرضى يكون على أحد أربعة أوجه : إمّا أن يأتي المريض بحران رديء تامّ الرداءة فيموت في يومه ذلك وإمّا أن تنحلّ قوة المريض قليلا قليلا حتى يموت ويسمّى ذبولا وإمّا أن يجمع الأمرين وهو أن ينقلب دفعة إلى الحال التي هي أردأ ثمّ لا يزال قوة المريض تذبل قليلا قليلا حتى يموت . وقد يموت العليل دفعة بلا بحران أصلا . ثالثة البحران .

١٠١ . قال موسى : معلوم أنّ هذا الموت دفعة دون بحران لا يمكن أن يكون في انحطاط المرض بل في أحد الثلاثة أوقات المتقدّمة للانحطاط . فإنّ جالينوس قد بيّن في ثالثة البحران ألا يقع الموت أصلا في انحطاط المرض إلا أن يموت من خطأ يعرض للمريض .

١٠٢ . كلّ مرض يسكن بغير استفراغ بيّن أو بخراج ذي قدر فإنّه يعاود بأخبث حال ممّا كان . ثالثة البحران .

١٠٣ . الذين يموتون بلا بحران ففي يوم النوبة يكون الموت . وقد يموت الواحد منهم في أوّل نوائب الحمّى وقد يموت في انتهاء النوبة وقد يموت في انحطاط النوبة عند انحلال القوة . ثالثة البحران .

١٠٤ . الأشياء كلّها التي تستفرغ من البدن إنّما تصير إلى الاستفراغ بضربين فمرّة يستفرغ من قبل الأجرام الحاوية لها تخرجها وتنفضها ومرّة يكون استفراغها لأنّ تلك

---

٤ أوجه] وجوه B || ٥ فيموت] فيحدث G || ٦ يجمع] يجتمع SGB || ١٠ فإنّ] قال G | جالينوس] ان add. G[1] | بيّن] فرتب EL || ١٢ استفراغ] ظاهر add. EL

these very secretions[185] flow out spontaneously, since the bodies containing them are too weak to keep and retain them. *De locis affectis* 6.[186]

(105) Take care not to prescribe laxatives at the beginning of tumors in the anus and surrounding area, and do not prescribe diuretics when a tumor begins to appear in the urinary bladder, penis, or kidneys. Similarly, do not induce menstruation when a tumor first appears in the uterus or vulva. When a tumor first appears in the throat, the upper part of the mouth, the tongue, [or anywhere else] inside the mouth, be careful not to prescribe a gargle. For, [doing so] while there are tumors in those places is similar to prescribing purgatives in the case of a tumor in the intestines, or diuretics in the case of [a tumor in] the urinary bladder, or emetics in the case of a tumor in the stomach or esophagus. *De methodo medendi* 13.[187]

(106) The application of cupping glasses is one of the strong means to attract that which is in the depths of the body and to eliminate tumors which have become hard and solid. This should be done only once the whole body has been evacuated, for, if one applies cupping glasses to a part of the body while the body is full, they attract the [superfluous] matter to this part. Therefore, one should apply them on the side furthest from the ailing part of the body so that the matter is attracted from that part to the opposite side, as we have established. *De methodo medendi* 13.[188]

(107) The application of cupping glasses to the neck on the occipital protuberance is one of the best means to prevent the [superfluous] matters from streaming toward the eye. But [one] should do so only after the whole body has been evacuated. *De methodo medendi* 13.[189]

(108) Remember that if one treats a part of the body with dissolving drugs while the body is full [of superfluities], it is more probable and likely that these drugs will attract [those superfluities] to that part and fill it [with them] than that they will evacuate them. Therefore, if [one] treats hot tumors and the like, [one] should not rely on the application of dissolving drugs until [one has] evacuated the whole body. *De methodo medendi* 13.[190]

الرطوبات أنفسها تجري وتخرج إذا كانت الأجرام الحاوية قد ضعفت حتى لا تضبطها ولا تمسكها . سادسة التعرّف .

١٠٥ . احذر أن تلين البطن في ابتداء أورام الدبر وما حوله ولا تدرّ البول إن ابتدأ حـدوث ورم في المثانة والإحليل والكليتين . ولا تحدر الحيض في ابتداء حدوث ورم في الرحم أو الفرج . فأمّا الحلق وأعلى الفم واللسـان وجميع ما في الفم متى ابتدأت أن ترم فاحذر الغرغرة . فإنّها في هذا الموضع شـبيهة بإسهال البطن عند ورم الأمعاء وإدرار البول عند ورم المثانة أو القيء عند تورّم المعدة والمريء . ثالثة عشرة الحيلة .

١٠٦ . تعليق المحاجم من الأشـياء القوية فـي اجتذاب ما في عمق البدن وقلع الأورام التي قد استحكمت صلابتها . ولا تفعل ذلك إلا بعد استفراغ البدن كلّه لأنّك إن علّقت المحجمة على العضو والبدن ممتلئ جذبت له المادّة . فإنّما تعلّقها على الجهة البعيـدة عن العضو العليل حتى تجذب المادّة عنه إلى خلاف الجهة كما أصّلنا . ثالثة عشرة الحيلة .

١٠٧ . إذا علّقت المحجمة على القفاء في موضع الفأس كانت من أقوى الأشياء نفعا في منع انصباب الموادّ إلى العين . ولا ينبغي أن تفعل ذلك إلا بعد استفراغ جملة البدن كلّه . ثالثة عشرة الحيلة .

١٠٨ . تذكر أنّ الأدوية المحلّلة إذا عولج بها عضو ما وكان في البدن امتلاء فهي إلى أن تجذب إلى العضو وتملأه أحرى وأقرب من أن تستفرغ . ولذلك إذا داويت الأورام الحارّة وغيرها لا تثق باستعمال المحلّلة حتى تستفرغ جملة البدن . ثالثة عشرة الحيلة .

---

١٣ موضع] om. B | الفأس] الرأس SL

(109) There are physicians who think that the stronger a medicine is in astringency, the more effective it is, when astringency is required. They also think that the more dispersing a medicine is, the more effective and beneficial it is, when dispersion is required. They do not understand that the stronger either of these powers is, the stronger the pain caused by it in the tumorous part of the body. The reason is that a very astringent medicine causes something similar to a contusion and disruption because the substance of the bodily part is severely drawn together and compressed, while hot medicines with a strongly dispersing action cause something similar to a corrosion in the tumorous part of the body. Truly, a medicine with a power intermediate between these two is better than [either] extreme one. *Mayāmir* 5.[191]

(110) Do not cool nor restrain the tumor of erysipelas until you have evacuated the entire body through purgation of the abdomen with a drug which expels the yellow bile. If you first chill and restrain and then evacuate [the body], it often happens that the erysipelas is driven from the organ in which it [resides] to a principal organ—and this is very dangerous. *De methodo medendi* 14.[192]

(111) The following matter is of great importance, and you must keep it in mind—namely, that a remedy composed with a certain goal and aim is often mixed with other ingredients which do not fit that goal, nor the intended use. But this remedy is mixed [with other ingredients] so that it will not cause any kind of pain or harm. *Mayāmir* 7.[193]

(112) Says Moses: In this way, mastic—an astringent remedy—is added to purgatives in order to strengthen the cardia of the stomach and to suppress the urge which is caused by purgatives to vomit and throw up. Similarly, gum tragacanth is added to prevent [possible] harm caused to the intestines by colocynth.

١٠٩. في الأطبّاء قوم يحسبون أنّ كلّ ما كان أشدّ قبضا فهو أبلغ في ما يراد به التقبيض. وكذلك ما كان من الأدوية أكثر تحليلا فهو أبلغ وأنفع في ما يراد تحليله. وليس يفهمون أنّ كلّ واحدة من هاتين القوّتين كلّ ما كانت أقوى كان ما يحدث عنها في العضو الوارم من الوجع أشدّ، لأنّ القابض بشدّة يحدث عنه شبيه بالرضّ والفسخ لأنّ جوهر العضو يجتمع ويكتنز اجتماعا عنيفا والأدوية الحارّة التي تحلّل تحليلا قويا يحدث عنها في العضو الوارم شيء شبيه بالتأكّل. فبالحقّ صار المعتدل في كلّ واحدة من هاتين القوّتين أفضل من المفرط. خامسة الميامر.

١١٠. لا تبرد ولا تردع ورم الحمرة حتى تستفرغ جملة البدن بإسهال البطن بدواء يخرج الصفراء. وإن تقدّمت بالتبريد والردع قبل الاستفراغ فكثير ما يدفع عن العضو الذي فيه الحمرة إلى عضو نفيس جليل الخطر. رابعة عشرة الحيلة.

١١١. هذا أمر عظيم جليل القدر جدّا ينبغي أن يكون حاضرا لذكرك وهو أن الدواء المؤلّف ليقصد به قصدا ما وغرضا ما كثيرا ما تخلط فيه أدوية آخر غير ملائمة لذلك الغرض وغير موافقة لمنفعته التي قصد به إليها. وإنّما نخلطها كيلا يؤلم ولا يوذي بوجه من الوجوه. سابعة الميامر.

١١٢. قال موسى: مثل ما يخلط المصطكى وهو دواء قابض مع المسهلات كي يقوّي فم المعدة ويمنع من تغثية المسهلات أو قذفها. وكما يخلط الكثيراء لمنع أذية شحم الحنظل بالمعى.

---

١ في الأطبّاء] om. B | به] فيه EL || ٥ نخلطها] نخالطها G

(113) If someone's humors are thin and fine, and if he is close to fainting because of the dissolution of the pneuma which necessarily follows from the thinness of the humors, and if he has a tumor in his liver or stomach, then there is absolutely no cure for him nor remedy: his strength has collapsed, and feeding him [in order to strengthen him] is impossible because of the tumor. *De methodo medendi* 12.[194]

(114) It is impossible to compose a single remedy that can cure all [ailing] bodies; for difference in temperaments of bodies and difference in ages makes a large variety in medicines necessary. For this reason, one should have two medicines ready: one stronger than all the [other] medicines of the same kind, and the other weaker than all the others. These one should mix according to the need [whenever one wishes]. *Qaṭājānas* 3.[195]

(115) Sweat is something unnatural, because, when the body functions properly and when nature overpowers and overcomes the food, sweat is not emitted. *In Hippocratis Aphorismos commentarius* 1.[196]

This is the end of the third treatise,
by the grace of God, praise be to Him.

◆

١١٣ . مـن كانت أخلاطه رقيقة لطيفة وقارب الغشـي من أجـل ما يلزم رقّة الأخلاط من تحلّل الروح وورمت كبده أو معدته فمرضه لا بروء له ولا دواء البتّة إذ كانت قوّتهم قد سقطت وامتنعت التغذية من أجل الورم. ثانية عشرة الحيلة.

١١٤ . ليس يمكن أن تؤلّف دواء واحدا يصلح به جميع الأبدان لأنّ اختلاف الأبدان في أمزجتها واختلاف الأسنان يوجب اختلافا كثيرا في الأدوية. وبهذا السبب ينبغي أن يكون عندك دواءان معدّان أحدهما أقوى من جميع الأدوية الداخلة في جنسه والدواء الآخر أضعفها كلّها. وتخلطها بحسب الحاجة متى شئت. ثالثة قطاجانس.

١١٥ . العـرق هو خـارج عن الطبيعة لأنّ أمر البـدن إذا جرى على ما ينبغي واستولت الطبيعـة على الغذاء وقهرتـه لم ينبعث العرق. في شـرحه للأولى من الفصول. تمّت المقالة الثالثة بحمد اللّه ومنّه.

---

٣ من أجل] لأجل S | ثانية] ثالثة SG || ٥ الأسنان] الإنسان B || ٨ هو] أمر add. L ||
١٠ تمّت المقالة الثالثة بحمد اللّه ومنّه] om. B : كملت المقالة الثالثة والحمد للّه تعالى وعدد فصولها مائة وعشرون فصلا L : كملت المقالة الثالثة P

In the name of God, the Merciful, the Compassionate
O Lord, make [our task] easy

The Fourth Treatise

Containing aphorisms concerning the pulse and the prognostic signs to be derived from it

(1) The existence of the pulse is vital and useful for two things. One of these, the most important, is the maintenance of the innate heat. The second is the generation of the pneuma.[1] *De pulsu* 13.[2]

(2) The meaning of [the concept] of rhythm[3] mentioned in the [different] types of the pulse is the ratio of the time of expansion [of the arteries] to the time of rest which follows, and also of the time of contraction [of the arteries] to the time of rest with follows. The proportion between these two times is without any doubt according to what is natural for each of the [different] ages [of man]. Sometimes it is according to its nature, and sometimes it is different.[4] *De pulsu magna* 1.[5]

بسم الله الرحمن الرحيم ربّ يسّر

المقالة الرابعة

تشتمل على فصول تتعلّق بالنبض والاستدلال به

١ . الحاجـة إلى كون النبض والانتفاع به هو لأمرين . أحدهما وهو أجلّها خطرا حفظ الحرارة الغريزية . الثاني توليد الروح . ثالثة عشرة النبض .

٢ . معنى الوزن المذكور في أجناس النبض هي المقايسـة بين زمان الانبساط مع زمان السكون الذي بعده وبين زمان الانقباض مع زمان السكون الذي بعده . فإنّ لهذين الزمانين أحدهما عند الآخر بلا شكّ نسبة ما طبيعية بحسب كلّ واحد من الأسنان . فقد توجد تلك النسـبة على طبيعتها وقد تختلـف . في الأولى من النبض الكبير .

---

١ بسـم الله الرحمن الرحيم ربّ يسّـر] om. LBP : بسم الله الرحمن الرحيم S || ٨ أحدهما] لأحدهما L || ٨–٩ ما . . . تلك النسبة] om. L

(3) Knowledge about the rhythm can be obtained through the strongest possible pulse [only]. In other types of pulse, the rhythm either cannot be grasped at all or is grasped far from correctly.[6] *De pulsu* 7.[7]

(4) A constant, truthful indicator of the strength of the [animal] faculty[8] is a strong, equal pulse, and, similarly, a great pulse. *De [curandi ratione per] venae sectionem.*[9]

(5) The pulse of a newborn child is extremely rapid and frequent, while the pulse of old people is extremely slow and rare.[10] The [pulses normal for] other ages [fall] between these two by gradation. In the prime of adolescence, the pulse is greatest and strongest. Its greatness and strength diminish gradually until, in old age, it is weakest and smallest. From the time of birth until the prime of adolescence, the pulse gradually increases in greatness and strength. *De pulsu* 11.[11]

(6) When rarity, weakness, or smallness of the pulse are at their absolute extreme, they are very dangerous, and those who have this pulse are in constant fear [for their lives]. This is not the case when greatness and strength [of the pulse] are at their maximum. When rapidity [of the pulse] is at its maximum, it is more safe and secure than when slowness is at its extreme. *De pulsu* 14.[12]

(7) A pulse that has an irregular inequality indicates that the cause of the inequality[13] shifts [from organ to organ] and is not stable. It may shift to an inferior organ, [so that] the patient is spared. But it may also shift to a noble organ, leading to the patient's death. Therefore, one cannot use the irregularity [of the inequality of the pulse] as a genuine prognostic sign. *De pulsu* 14.[14]

٣ . تعرّف الوزن إنّما يكون إدراكه في النبض الشديد غاية الشدّة. وما سوى ذلك من النبض فإنّ الوزن لا يدرك فيه البتّة أو يدرك إدراكا بعيدا عن الحقيقي. سابعة النبض.

٤ . الدليل الذي يدلّ على شدّة القوة دائما ولا يكذب هو النبض القوي المستوي وكذلك النبض العظيم. في مقالته في الفصد.

٥ . الصغير عندما يولد نبضه في غاية السرعة والتواتر ونبض الشيوخ في غاية البطء والتفاوت. وسائر الأسنان في ما بين ذلك على التدريج. وفي سنّ غاية الشباب يكون النبض أعظم ما يكون وأقواه. وينقص العظم والقوة على التدريج حتى يكون في سنّ الشيخ أضعف ما يكون وأصغره. وأمّا من حين الولادة إلى منتهى الشباب فإنّ النبض يزداد عظما وقوة علي التدريج. حادية عشرة النبض.

٦ . تفاوت النبض أو ضعفه أو صغره كلّ واحد من هذه الثلاثة أصناف إذا كان في الغاية التي ليست وراءها غاية فإنّها مخوفة جدّا وأصحابه على وجل دائما. وليس العظم والقوة في الغاية كذلك. أمّا السرعة في الغاية فإنّها آمن وأسلم من الأبطأ في الغاية. رابعة عشرة النبض.

٧ . النبض المختلف اختلاف غير منتظم يدلّ على أنّ سبب الاختلاف منتقل غير ثابت. فقد تنتقل العلّة إلى عضو خسيس فيتخلّص المريض أو ينتقل إلى عضو شريف فيهلك المريض. فليس يستدلّ إذا من خلاف النظام على شيء حقيقي. رابعة عشر النبض.

١–١٠ تعرّف . . . عاشرة النبض (at bk. 4, sec. 11) [om. E || ٢ فيه] om. B : النسبة add. G || ٩ الشيخ] الشيوخ LB || ١٣ من الأبطأ] والالأبطأ G || ١٧ خلاف] خارج L

(8) A regular unequal pulse [that adheres to one pattern] indicates that the cause of the inequality is stable and fixed. When it is the opposite of this, it is neither stable nor fixed. *De pulsu* 10.[15]

(9) All the types of pulse which are unequal in more than one beat are the necessary result either of an irregular temperament of the heart or of an affliction occurring to the organ[16] or to the faculty. *De pulsu* 10.[17]

(10) When the faculty is weak in itself, it rarely makes a pulse unequal in its beats. But if the faculty is powerful in itself and is then burdened by a large amount of humors, the pulse becomes unequal in its beats. *De pulsu* 10.[18]

(11) The first and lowest degree of weakness of the faculty makes the pulse smaller and fainter. The next degree of weakness is that in which one's fingers put on the artery are a burden for the faculty. It turns one's pulse into the recurrent[19] one called "mouse tail."[20] When the faculty is wasted and dissolved [even] more than this, it turns one's pulse into the permanent "mouse tail." *De pulsu* 10.[21]

(12) A strong pulse always strikes a forceful beat. Similarly, a hard type of pulse strikes a forceful beat just like the vibratory and spasmodic pulses.[22] *De pulsu* 8.[23]

(13) One never finds that the same pulse is very hard and at the same time very great. One also never finds that the same pulse is very great or very strong and at the same time slow. But in most cases [one finds] that the pulse which is very great is rapid and not slow. *De pulsu* 5. [24]

(14) The pulse that is great, very strong, and hard, and, to the same extent, the pulse that combines hardness with extreme greatness, has a contraction that is clearer and more evident than that of any other pulse.[25]

٨. النبــض المختلف اللازم لطريق واحدة يدلّ على أنّ ســبب الاختلاف ثابت متمكّن. وفي خلافه غير ثابت ولا متمكّن. عاشرة النبض.

٩. جميع أصناف النبض المختلف في أكثر من نبضة واحدة إنّما يتبع ويلزم سوء مزاج القلب المختلف أو الآفة الحادثة بالآلة أو بالقوة. عاشرة النبض.

١٠. القوة متى كانت ضعيفة في نفسها فقلّ أن تجعل النبض مختلفا في نبضات. أمّا متى كانت القوة في نفســها قوية وأثقلتها كثــرة الأخلاط فإنّ النبض يختلف في نبضاته. عاشرة النبض.

١١. أوّل مراتــب ضعف القوة وأقلّهــا يجعل النبض أزيد صغرا وأزيد خمولا. والمرتبة التي تتلو هذه في ضعفها هي التي تجعله يثقلها معه وضع الأصابع التي توضع على العرق. وتجعل النبض المســمّى ذنب الفــأرة العائد مرّة ثانية. وإن انتهكت القوة وانحلّت أكثر من هذا جعلت النبض ذنب الفأرة الثابت. عاشرة النبض.

١٢. النبض الشديد يقرع أبدا قرعا عنيفا. وكذلك نوع النبض الصلب يقرع قرعا عنيفا بمنزلة النبض المرتعد والنبض المتواتر. ثامنة النبض.

١٣. لا يوجــد أبدا نبضا واحدا بعينه صلبا جدّا عظيما جدّا معا. ولا يوجد أيضــا نبضا واحدا بعينه عظيما جدّا شــديدا جدّا بطيئــا. لكنّك تجد النبض أكثر النبض العظيم جدّا سريعا وغير بطيئا. خامسة النبض.

١٤. النبض الذي يجمع أن يكون عظيما شــديدا جدّا صلبا بقدر ما يمكن أن توجــد الصلابة مع العظم جدّا فإنّ انقباض هــذا النبض يكون أبين وأظهر من كلّ ما

---

١ الاختلاف] الغير اختلاف B ‖ ٢ بالآلة] به L ‖ ٩ يثقلها] تنقلها B : بنقله P | معه] .om L ‖ ١٠ مرّة] بعد add. P ‖ ١٤ يوجد] تجد ELBP

The contraction of the faint pulse is unknown. There is no way to detect or perceive it, either in the beginning of the movement of the expansion or in the end of the movement of the contraction. *De pulsu* 5.[26]

(15) Every disease that changes the pulse into a spasmodic one, if it lasts and becomes more severe and more difficult, changes the pulse into a vermicular one. Every disease that changes the pulse into a rare one, if it becomes more severe and more serious and lasts for a long time, makes the pulse unequal, and it seems as if the body of the artery has fragmented and broken into separate, small pieces. *De pulsibus libellus [ad tirones].*[27]

(16) Inequality [of the pulse] is in most cases accompanied by irregularity; one hardly ever finds a regular unequal pulse. When an affliction is minor, it turns the pulse into a regular unequal one; and, when it is major, it turns the pulse into an irregular unequal one. *De pulsibus libellus [ad tirones].*[28]

(17) When the faculty is dissolved, it makes the pulse small, weak, and very spasmodic. When it is oppressed and burdened, it turns the pulse into an irregular unequal one. The greater the affliction, the more the different kinds of variation [in pulse], especially in [its] strength and greatness. Inequality is in most cases followed by irregularity [of the pulse]. *De pulsibus libellus [ad tirones].*[29]

(18) Sometimes the temperament of the heart is warmer than is necessary and the temperament of the arteries colder than is necessary, or the reverse. Similarly, the body of the heart itself is sometimes cooler than its natural temperament,[30] while the substance contained in the two ventricles of the heart is warmer; or the reverse [may occur], in which case the pulse is similar to the natural pulse. These kinds of illnesses[31] lead astray [even] skilled physicians—let alone other physicians—and cause them to commit mistakes. *De pulsu* 15.[32]

سواه. وأمّا النبض الخامل فانقباضه مجهول لا يعرف ولا يحسّ منه بوجه بمبدأ حركة الانبساط ولا بنهاية حركة الانقباض. خامسة النبض.

١٥. كلّ مرض يغيّر النبض للمتواتر فإنّه إذا تطاول واشتدّ واستصعب جعل النبض دوديا. وكلّ مرض يغيّر النبض إلى التفاوت فإنّه مع زيادته وتطاوله وشدّته يجعل للنبض اختلافا يوهم أنّ جرم العرق قد تفتّت حتى صار العرق أجزاء صغار غير متّصلة. في النبض الصغير.

١٦. الاختلاف في أكثر الحالات يلزمه سوء النظام ولا تكاد تجد نبضا مختلفا منتظما إلا في الندرة. ومتى كانت الآفة يسيرة جعلت النبض مختلفا منتظما ومتى كانت الآفة عظيمة جعلت النبض مختلفا غير منتظما. النبض الصغير.

١٧. متى انحلّت القوة جعلت النبض صغيرا ضعيفا متواترا جدّا. ومتى ضغطها شيء وأثقلها جعلت النبض مختلفا غير منتظما. وكلّما كانت الآفة أعظم كانت أصناف الاختلاف أكثر وبخاصّة الاختلاف في القوة والعظم. والاختلاف في الأكثر يتبعه سوء النظام. في مقالته في النبض الصغير.

١٨. قد يكون مزاج القلب أسخن ممّا ينبغي ومزاج العروق الضوارب أبرد ممّا ينبغي وبالعكس. وكذلك القلب نفسه يتّفق كم مرّة أن يكون جرم القلب أبرد من مزاجه الطبيعي ويكون الجوهر الذي تحتوي عليه تجويفاه أحرّ وبالعكس ويكون النبض شبيها بالنبض الطبيعي. وأمثال هذه العلل تضلّ وتغلط حذّاق الأطبّاء فضلا عن غيرهم. خامسة عشرة النبض.

---

٧ تكاد تجد] يكاد يوجد EL || ٩ مختلفا] om. S || ١٦ تجويفاه] تجاويفه EL : نحو مزاج add. S

(19) A bad humor often collects in the cardia of the stomach and burns it or cools it, [so that] the pulse becomes small and unequal. The difference between burning and cooling is that the pulse becomes smaller as a result of cooling and it becomes more unequal as a result of burning. *De [differentiis] febrium* 1.[33]

(20) When biting, pain, pressure, vomiting, fainting, or hiccups occur at the cardia of the stomach, the pulse becomes very spasmodic, small, and weak, and sometimes also rapid. When the cardia of the stomach is compressed or squeezed by a large amount of food or by nonbiting humors streaming to it, the pulse becomes rare, slow, small, and weak. *De pulsu parva.*[34]

(21) If a [varying] bad temperament occurs in an artery,[35] that part of it containing more moisture and heat has a pulse that is greater and more rapid, whereas the part which is either cold or dry has a pulse that is smaller and slower. *De pulsu* 10.[36]

(22) In the beginning of all the putrefying fevers, the contraction of the artery is more rapid. This is a very reliable[37] diagnostic sign. [One] should rely on it as a prognostic sign more than on any other sign. A similar thing happens to the pulse when the attacks [of these fevers] are increasing and intensifying. And, when they reach the state of their culmination, the movements of contraction and expansion of the pulse are [less][38] rapid. *De pulsu* 15.[39]

(23) If at any time during the beginning of a fever you find the pulse strong and great but not hard, that fever is not a hectic fever under any circumstances. For, when the pulse is strong and great but not hard, it is a clear sign that it is an ephemeral fever. But, when you find the pulse weak and small and the artery hard, it is a hectic fever. *De pulsu* 15.[40]

(24) If much cold matter reaches the heart during the beginning of a fever attack, the patient is in a state close to death. This state is indicated

١٩ . كثيــرا ما يجتمع في فــم المعدة خلط رديء فيلذعه أو يبرده فيصير النبض صغيرا مختلفا . وممّا يميّز به ما يلذع ممّا يبرد أن صغر النبض الحادث من الشيء المبرد أكثر واختلاف النبض الحادث من الشيء الملذع أزيد . في الأولى من الحمّايات .

٢٠ . إذا حدث في فم المعدة لذع أو توجّع أو كرب أو قيء أو غشــي أو فواق فإنّ النبض يصير متواترا جدّا صغيرا ضعيفا وربّما صار ســريعا أيضا . ومتى ضغط فم المعدة أو عصره كثرة الطعام أو أخلاط غير لذّاعة انصبّت له فيصير النبض متفاوتا بطيئا صغيرا ضعيفا . في النبض الصغير .

٢١ . إذا كان في العرق سوء مزاج مختلف فإنّ الجزء منه الأكثر رطوبة وحرارة يكون نبضه أعظم وأسرع والجزء منه الذي يكون إمّا باردا أو يابسا يكون نبضه أصغر وأبطأ . عاشرة النبض .

٢٢ . فــي ابتداء حمّيات العفونة كلّها يكون انقباض العرق أزيد ســرعة . وهذه علامة بعيدة جدّا عن الكذب . وينبغي أن تثق بها في باب التعرّف أكثر من ثقتك بكلّ علامــة أخرى . وكذلك أيضا يكون النبض في تزيّد تلك النوائب وصعودها . أمّا في حال انتهائها فإنّ حركة الانقباض والانبساط سريعتين . خامسة عشرة النبض .

٢٣ . متى وجدت في وقت من الأوقات في ابتداء الحمّى النبض قويا أو عظيما أو عريا عن الصلابة فليســت تلك الحمّى حمّــى دقّ بوجه . ومتى كان النبض قويا عظيمــا عادم الصلابــة فذلك دلالة بيّنة على أنّها حمّى يــوم . ومتى وجدت النبض ضعيفا صغيرا والعرق صلبا فهي حمّى دقّ . خامسة عشرة النبض .

٢٤ . إذا صــارت مــادّة باردة كثيرة إلــى القلب في وقت ابتــداء نوبة الحمّى فــإنّ العليل فــي حال يشــرف فيها على المــوت . ويــدلّ على ذلك تغيّــر النبض

---

٣ أزيد] أكثر صرعا L

by a tremendous change of the pulse into rarity, slowness, and smallness. So, when these three [conditions] are followed by considerable[41] weakness, the patient will die instantly. *De pulsu* 15.[42]

(25) The arteries which are closest to the diseased organ undergo the greatest change into softness or hardness [of the pulse]. The arteries which are far from the diseased organ do not change unless the heart mediates between them and the diseased organ.[43] *De pulsu* 16.[44]

(26) When the pulse beat of all the arteries is weak, the animal faculty is weak in itself because of the [bad] temperament of the body of the heart, as is well known. When it is [weak] in one organ of the body, that organ alone is the one with a bad temperament. If the same artery sometimes has a weak pulse beat and sometimes a strong one, the [animal] faculty is not weak in itself but is burdened and strangled by a large amount of [superfluous] matter. *De pulsu* 16.[45]

(27) When the body of the heart itself becomes excessively cold or warm or moist or dry, in proportion to a bad temperament occurring to it, it makes the pulse weak and is an affliction affecting the faculty of the heart itself. When the blood and pneuma contained within the heart become hot or cold, or when the body of the pericardium or the body of the lung become hot or cold and that bad temperament passes to the heart but does not lodge in its body, nothing more happens than the necessary change [in the pulse]. The affliction does not affect the faculty [of the heart]. *De pulsu* 13.[46]

(28) When the blood or the pneuma enclosed by the body of the heart or the body of the pericardium or the lung change their temperament to dryness or moistness, [their pulse] does not necessarily change from what it was, because only heat and cold cause a necessary change. *De pulsu* 13.[47]

مقدارا كثيرا جدّا إلى التفاوت والإبطاء والصغر. فإن تبع هذه الثلاثة ضعف ذو قدر يعتدّ به مات العليل من ساعته. خامسة عشرة النبض.

٢٥. العروق التي هي من العضو العليل أقرب فهي أكثر تغيّرا إلى اللين والصلابة. وأمّا العروق البعيدة عن العضو العليل فلا تتغيّر إلا بواسطة القلب بينها وبين العضو العليل. سادسة عشرة النبض.

٢٦. متى كان نبض العروق كلّها ضعيفا فالقوة الحيوانية ضعيفة في نفسها بسبب مزاج جرم القلب كما علم. وإن كان ذلك في عضو واحد من البدن فإنّ ذلك العضو وحده هو الذي ساء مزاجه. ومتى كان عرق واحد بعينه مرّة نبضه ضعيفا ومرّة قويا فليست القوة ضعيفة في نفسها لكنّ هناك مادّة كثيرة قد ثقلت على القوة وخنقتها. سادسة عشرة النبض.

٢٧. متى برد جرم القلب نفسه أو سخن أو رطب أو يبس بإفراط بحسب ما يصير عليه من سوء المزاج يجعل النبض ضعيفا وهذا هو وقوع الآفة بقوة القلب نفسه. أمّا متى سخن أو برد الدم والروح اللّذان يحويهما القلب أو سخن أو برد جرم غلاف القلب أو جرم الرئة وتعدّى ذلك سوء المزاج إلى القلب ولم يستحكم في جرمه فليس يحدث شيء أكثر من تغيّر الحاجة فقط خلوا من وقوع الآفة بالقوة. ثالثة عشرة النبض.

٢٨. إن كان الدم والروح اللّذان يحويهما جرم القلب أو جرم غلاف القلب أو الرئة تغيّر مزاجها لليبس أو للرطوبة فليس تتغيّر الحاجة عمّا كانت عليه فإنّ الحرّ والبرد فقط هما اللّذان يغيّران الحاجة. ثالثة عشرة النبض.

---

١ مقدارا كثيرا] بمقدار كثير ELP

(29) In most conditions of a crisis [of a disease], the arterial pulse is unequal, especially when the crisis goes with severe exhaustion.[48] When the pulse is hard, it indicates vomiting. When the pulse is undulatory,[49] it indicates sweat; when it is great but not undulatory, it indicates a hemorrhage,[50] [because it indicates] a movement of nature toward the outside of the body through blood streaming from the nose or from other places. A high pulse and a strong pulse during a crisis are both[51] signs of all kinds of evacuation. *De crisibus* 3.[52]

(30) When the heat of the body increases, the pulse changes first of all toward greatness. When the heat increases further, the pulse increases in rapidity together with greatness. When the heat increases even more than that, the pulse becomes more rapid and greater and also more spasmodic. When the body cools off, the first thing that can be noticed about the pulse is rarity, followed by slowness, and then, in the third place, by smallness. *De pulsu* 10.[53]

(31) When the arteries are surrounded by things which press upon them and occupy the places of their expansion, be these things humors or tumors, the pulse beats will be unequal. Similarly, a large amount of blood discharged into the arteries or veins can make the pulse unequal in the same way. In general, where some sort of heavy pressure or of blockage happens to the arteries, the pulse will be unequal in its beat. *De pulsu* 10.[54]

(32) Softness of an organ causes greatness of the pulse, and the domination of cold over the body causes smallness [of the pulse]. Sometimes the degree of smallness caused by the cold and [the degree] of greatness caused by the softness of the organ are similar, so that the pulse stays moderate.

٢٩ . نبض العرق في أكثر حالات البحران يكون مختلفا ولا سيّما إذا كان مع البحران جهد عظيم . وإن كان النبض صلبا دلّ على القيء . والنبض الموجي يدلّ على العرق والعظيم الغير الموجي يدلّ على الدم لأنّه يدلّ على حركة الطبيعة لظاهر البدن بدم يجري من المنخرين أو غيرهما . والنبض المشرف والقوي علامة مشتركة في البحران لجميع أنحاء الاستفراغ. ثالثة البحران.

٣٠ . إذا تزيّدت حرارة البدن فأوّل ما يتغيّر النبض إلى العظم . فإن زادت الحرارة على تلك ازداد مع العظم سرعة . فإن زادت على هذه أيضا ازداد معهما التواتر . فأمّا إذا برد البدن فأوّل ما يتبيّن في النبض التفاوت ويتلو التفاوت الإبطاء والثالث بعدهما الصغر . تاسعة النبض .

٣١ . العروق الضوارب إذا أحاط بها أشياء تضغطها وتشغل مواضع انبساطها سواء كانت تلك الأشياء أخلاطا أو أوراما فإنّ النبض يختلف نبضاته . وكذلك كثرة الدم المفرغ في العروق الضوارب أو غير الضوارب قد تجعل النبض مختلفا هذا الاختلاف . وبالجملة متى عرض للعروق الضوارب ما يزحمها زحما شديدا أو يسدّها فإنّ النبض يكون مختلفا في نبضه . عاشر النبض .

٣٢ . لين الآلة يوجب العظم في النبض وغلبة البرودة على البدن توجب الصغر . وقد يكون ما يوجبه البرد من الصغر مثل ما يوجبه لين الآلة من العظم فيبقى معتدلا . وكذلك كل سببين مختلفين متكافة القوة من الأسباب المغيّرة للنبض يكون النبض من

---

٤ مشتركة] مشهورة EL || ٥ البحران] البحارين ELBP || ٦–٧ الحرارة . . . زادت] om. EL || ١٠ أحاط] أحس L || ١١–١٢ نبضاته . . . تجعل النبض] om. E || ١٢ المفرغ] المفرط L || ١٨ سببين] شيئين B | متكافة] متكافي L : مكتفين E : متكافين B

Similarly, if each of the two causes which change the pulse are equal in strength, the pulse will be moderate. In the case of someone who is ill and in this condition, one might think that his pulse is still in its natural condition. However, this is not so, because every natural pulse is moderate between two extremes, but not every moderate pulse is natural. *De pulsu* 9.[55]

(33) As the undulatory pulse, when it becomes small and light and little, is followed by the vermicular one, so the vermicular pulse, when most of its motions stop and only one motion is left, is followed by the antlike pulse, which is a very small motion similar to the crawling of an ant. It is actually unequal, but because it is so small the senses cannot distinguish its inequality. This pulse is extremely small, weak, and spasmodic; there is no pulse which is smaller, weaker, or more spasmodic. One may think that it is rapid, but it is not rapid [in reality]. *De pulsu* 1.[56]

(34) The dissolution of the faculty is in most cases followed first by the vermicular pulse and then by the antlike [pulse]. When the faculty is dissolved without fever or with a light fever, it is especially followed by the vermicular [pulse], and it remains [so] for a long time. *De pulsibus libellus [ad tirones].*[57]

(35) Sometimes the pulse hardens in the case of ephemeral fever, putrefying fever, or hectic fever; this is caused by one of those things which harden the pulse, but not by the fever. For fever itself—in its capacity of fever—does not necessarily accompany a hard pulse under all circumstances. But the pulse is in most cases found to be hard in the case of hectic fever. *De [differentiis] febrium* 1.[58]

One may think that the pulse of those suffering from spasms[59] is strong and great, while in reality it is neither weak, nor strong, nor small, nor great. Its tension may give the impression of strength,[60] and because of its trembling motion one may imagine that it jumps and rises very much.[61] *De pulsu.*[62]

أجلهما معتدلا. فيظــنّ بمن كانت هذه حاله في مرضه أنّه باق على حاله الطبيعية. وليــس الأمــر كذلك لأنّ كلّ نبض طبيعي معتدل بين الطرفــين وليس كلّ نبض معتدل طبيعيا. تاسعة النبض.

٣٣. كمــا يعقب النبض الموجــي إذا صغر وقلّ النبض الــدودي كذلك يعقب الدودي إذا بطلت حركاته الكثيرة وبقيت فيه حركة واحدة النبض النملي وهي حركة قليلة جدّا شــبيهة بدبيب النمل. وفيــه بالحقيقة اختلاف لكن لصغره لا يدرك الحسّ اختلافــه. وهذا النبض في غاية الصغر والضعف والتواتر ولا يوجد نبض أصغر ولا أضعف ولا أشدّ تواترا منه. ويوهم السرعة وليس بسريع. أولى النبض.

٣٤. انحلال القوة يتبعه في أكثر الأمر أوّلا النبض الدودي ثمّ بآخره يتبعه النملي. ومتى انحلّت القوة من غير حمّى أو مع حمّى يسيرة تبعه الدودي خاصّة ويثبت زمانا طويلا. النبض الصغير.

٣٥. قــد يصلب النبض مع حمّى يوم أو مع الحمّى العفنية أو مع حمّى الدقّ من أحد الأســباب المصلّبة للنبض لا من أجل الحمّى. لأنّ نفس الحمّى من طريق ما هي حمّى فليس يلزم عنها في حال من الأحوال صلابة النبض إلا أنّه أكثر ما يوجد النبض صلبا مع حمّى الدقّ. في الأولى من الحمّيات.

يوهم نبض أصحاب التشنّج أنّه قوي عظيم وأمّا بالحقيقة فليس هو ضعيف ولا قوي ولا صغير ولا عظيم. وإنّما تمدّده يوهم القوّة ويخيّل برعدة حركته أنّه يثب ويرتفع كثيرا. النبض الصغير.

---

١٠ من] مع ELBP || ١٣ أحد] أجل S

(36) Internal rest [of the artery] can never be known for certain, but it is possible to perceive it by means of firm palpation when the pulse is very strong. *De pulsu* 5.[63]

Do not palpate an artery firmly in any kind of pulse, except for the strong pulse only. But also in this case, [one should] not palpate so firmly that the strength [of the artery] is overwhelmed. *De pulsu* 5.[64]

(37) When the faculty is powerful and the body of the artery is hard and the need is urgent,[65] the pulse will be vibratory. When one of these [factors] is missing, the pulse will not be vibratory. *De pulsu* 10.[66]

(38) When the faculty becomes very weak, not only does it make the pulse weak, but also small and, because of its smallness, dense.[67] When the faculty becomes powerful, it makes the pulse strong and great; if the need does not change at all, [it also makes it very rare].[68] *De pulsu* 13.[69]

(39) The vermicular pulse is caused by weakness of the faculty. The undulatory pulse is caused by an excess of moisture and sometimes by extreme softness of the organ.[70] *De pulsu* 10.[71]

(40) Something that every unequal pulse has in common is that it is caused either by obstructions, or by pressure which occurs to an organ, or by an amount of humors greater than the measure of the faculty, or [by] an unequal bad temperament of the heart. Inequality in one [kind of] pulse is more serious and difficult than when it occurs in many [kinds of] pulses.[72] A weak pulse does not indicate anything other than a bad temperament of the heart. It is only necessarily followed by inequality [of the pulse] when it is joined by one of the three [other] causes mentioned previously. *De pulsu* 14.[73]

٣٦ . السكون الداخل لا يمكن تعرّفه يقينا في وقت من الأوقات . لكنّه قد يدرك إذا كان النبض شديدا جدّا وغمزت عليه غمزا عنيفا . خامسة النبض .

لا تغمز على العرق في صنف من أصناف النبض إلا في النبض الشديد وحده . ولا تغمز عليه أيضا غمزا عنيفا تقهر به القوة . خامسة النبض .

٣٧ . إذا كانت القوة قوية وجرم العرق صلبا والحاجة تدعو كثيرا كان النبض مرتعدا . ومتى نقصت واحدة من هذه فليس يكون النبض مرتعدا . عاشرة النبض .

٣٨ . القوة التي قد ضعفت ضعفا كثيرا ليس تصيّر النبض ضعيفا فقط بل تجعله أيضا صغيرا ومن أجل صغره تجعله متواترا . ومتى قويت القوة جعلت النبض مع قوّته عظيما وإن كانت الحاجة لم تتغيّر بتّة . ثالثة عشرة النبض .

٣٩ . السبب في النبض الدودي ضعف القوة . وفي النبض الموجي إفراط الرطوبة وقد يكون في بعض الأوقات بسبب لين الآلة في الغاية القصوى . عاشرة النبض .

٤٠ . الشيء العامّ لكلّ نبض مختلف هو أنّه يكون بسبب سدد أو ضغط يعرض للآلة أو أخلاط تكثر عن مقدار القوة أو سوء مزاج مختلف يعرض للقلب . والاختلاف في نبضة واحدة أشدّ وأصعب من كونه في نبضات كثيرة . والنبض الضعيف ليس هو دليل شيء آخر خلاء سوء مزاج القلب . وليس يلزم عن ضعفه اختلاف إلا أن ينضاف إلى ذلك أحد الثلاثة الأسباب التي ذكرناها الآن . رابعة عشرة النبض .

---

٦ ومتى . . . عاشرة النبض] om. B || ٧ ضعفا] قويا add. S || ١٥ خلاء] خلاف EL

(41) Ascites is caused by moisture collecting in the abdomen, whereby the vessels widen and cool off. In this case, the pulse tends toward hardness and becomes small and dense,[74] especially when it is accompanied by fever. Anasarca[75] makes the pulse undulatory because it moistens all the hard organs[76] of the body and soaks them.[77] *De pulsu* 12.[78]

(42) I do not know anyone who was saved from pleurisy when his pulse was extremely hard, small, and very dense. *De pulsu* 16.[79]

(44)[80] Do not imagine the movement of the artery in three dimensions as a movement in a cubic body or a cone or a similar body, but think of it as a singular movement and a singular rotation, as the movement of a sphere; for the movement of the artery as it appears to the senses is that of a perfect rotation. *De pulsu* 7.[81]

(45) The pulse is never extremely slow and small as long as the faculty is strong, even if the need [for it] has become extremely slight. *De pulsu* 9.[82]

(46) A pulse with a double beat[83] is sometimes caused by an extremely bad temperament and a slight hardness of an artery, and sometimes by extreme hardness [of an artery] with weakness of the faculty,[84] or thickness and abundance of the humors. *De pulsu* 10.[85]

(47) The pulse is natural[86] when the faculty is in a balanced condition[87] and protected from being moved by either an excessive fullness of the organ[88] or its obstruction or compression by something [else]. *De pulsu* 10.[89]

(48) An unequal bad temperament of the organ[90] makes the pulse fragmented.[91] *De pulsu* 12.[92]

This is the end of the fourth treatise
by the grace of God, praise be to Him.

◆

٤١ . الاستسقاء الزقّي من قبل ما يجتمع في البطن من الرطوبة فتتمدّد العروق وتبرد . فيصير النبض مائلا إلى الصلابة صغيرا متواترا ولا سيّما مع الحمّى . وأمّا الاستسقاء اللحمي فلكونه يبلّ أعضاء البدن الصلبة كلّها وينقعها يجعل النبض موجيا . ثانية عشرة النبض .

٤٢ . لا أعلم أحدا نجا من ذات الجنب إذا كان نبض صاحبها صلب غاية الصلابة صغيرا متواترا جدّا . سادسة عشرة النبض .

٤٤ . لا تتخيّل حركة العرق في ثلاثة أقطاره كحركته في الجسم المربّع أو المخروط وغيرهما بل تتوهّم أنّها حركة واحدة واستدارة واحدة كحركة الكرة لأنّ حركة العرق تتبيّن للحسّ مستديرة محكمة الاستدارة . سابعة النبض .

٤٥ . لا يكون النبض بتّة في غاية البطؤ والصغر ما دامت القوة قوية وإن كانت الحاجة قد قلّت غاية القلّة . تاسعة النبض .

٤٦ . النبض ذو القرعتين مرّة يكون من سوء مزاج عظيم وصلابة يسيرة في العرق ومرّة يكون عن صلابة عظيمة وضعف قوة أو مع غلظ وكثرة أخلاط . عاشرة النبض .

٤٧ . النبض الطبيعي يكون إذا كانت القوة على حال اعتدال وامتنعت من الحركة من قبل امتلاء مفرط أو سدّة أو ضغط شيء للآلة . عاشرة النبض .

٤٨ . سوء مزاج الآلة المختلف يجعل النبض متفتّتا . ثانية عشرة النبض . تمّت المقالة الرابعة ولله الحمد والمنّة .

---

١ الرطوبة] الرطوبات S || ٥ نجا] سلم EL || ٩ النبض] الفصول] G || ١٣ عن] من ELBP || ١٤ الطبيعي] البطيL : الطبي BGP || ١٦ تمّت المقالة الرابعة ولله الحمد والمنّة] om. B : كملت المقالة الرابعة وعدد فصولها تسعة وأربعون فصلا EL : كملت المقالة الرابعة P

In the name of God, the Merciful, the Compassionate
O Lord, make [our task] easy

The Fifth Treatise

Containing aphorisms concerning the [prognostic] signs to be derived from the urine

(1) In all the fevers, one should above all examine and inspect the urine, because fevers are illnesses in the veins.[1] In the case of pleurisy, one should first of all inspect the sputum and then the urine, because pleurisy does not occur without fever. When there is an illness in the abdomen accompanied by fever, one should first of all inspect the excrements and then the urine; and, if there is no fever, [one should] examine only the excrements. *De crisibus* 1.[2]

(2) The best sediment which descends with the urine in the case of putrefying fevers is that which comes from the putrefying humor when it is cocted in the vessel containing it. The resulting sediment which settles in the urine is white, smooth, and even and has a smell which is not unpleasant. *De [differentiis] febribum* 1.[3]

بسم اللّه الرحمن الرحيم ربّ يسّر

المقالة الخامسة

تشتمل على فصول تتعلّق بالاستدلال

١ . ينبغي في جميع الحمّيات أن يكون أكثر ما تفتقده وتنظر فيه البول إذ الحمّيات مرض في العروق . أمّا في ذات الجنب فتنظر أوّلا في النفث ثمّ تنظر بعد ذلك في البول إذ لا تنفكّ ذات الجنب عن حمّى . ومتى كان المرض في البطن وكان معه حمّى فتنظر أوّلا في البراز ثمّ تنظر في البول وإن لم يكن حمّى فتفقد البراز وحده . أولى البحران .

٢ . الثفل الذي ينحدر مع البول في الحمّيات التي من العفونة أجوده وهو الذي يكون من الخلط الذي قد عفن إذا أنضجه العرق الذي يحويه . يكون منه في البول ثفل راسب أبيض أملس مستوي غير كريه الرائحة . أولى الحمّيات .

---

١ بسم اللّه . . . ربّ يسّر] om. LBP : بسم اللّه الرحمن الرحيم وللّه الحمد S || ٦ تنفكّ] تنقل S(?) || ٧ وإن . . . البحران] om. B

(3) If the parts of the urine are all even in color and consistency, it indicates the domination and supremacy of nature over the illness.[4] When [bubbles of gassy] spirit accumulate in the urine, it is [caused by] a cold humor and therefore indicates that the illness will be prolonged.[5] *In Hippocratis Aphorismos commentarius* 7.[6]

(4) The best urine in ill people is that which is most similar to the urine of healthy people. The urine which has been cocted extremely well and which comes from someone who is extremely healthy is the urine which is even in its thickness and tends toward yellowness with a little bit of redness. It tends more to being completely yellow, as [is the case] if one were to take water and mix it with some of the watery part of the blood and yellow bile. *De crisibus* 1.[7]

(5) The best kind of urine is that which has a good color and a cloud which is white, smooth, and even. If [the cloud] settles to the bottom of a bottle, it is the best; if it is suspended in the middle, it is second best; and if it floats on the urine, it is third best.[8] These are the three kinds which indicate coction. Of all the other kinds of urine which remain, some indicate the opposite of coction,[9] and others indicate death.[10] *De crisibus* 1.[11]

(6) The evenness of a sediment is subject to two [kinds of] conditions. The first is that it should not be scattered and dispersed but combined, and the second that it should remain so all the time. For sometimes one finds the urine clear at one time but with a sediment at another time, and a laudable sediment does not appear continuously. This is a sign that the coction was not completed.[12] *De crisibus* 1.[13]

(7) The best urine of ill people is that which, when excreted, shows a laudable sediment with perfect characteristics, for this indicates that nature has overcome the illness and has begun to expel the humor causing the illness. The second-best urine is that which is turbid when it is excreted but in which, shortly after its excretion, a laudable sediment is deposited,

٣ . إذا كانت أجزاء البول كلّها متساوية في اللون والقوام دلّ ذلك على غلبة الطبيعة للمرض واستيلائها عليه . والذي يجمع الريح في البول هو الخلط البارد ولذلك يدلّ على طول من المرض . في شرحه لسابعة الفصول .

٤ . أفضل أبوال المرضى أشبه ببول الأصحّاء . والبول الناضج في الغاية ممّن هو في غاية الصحّة هو البول المعتدل الثخين الذي يضرب إلى الصفرة والحمرة اليسيرة . وهو إلى الأصفر المشبع أميل كما لو أخذت ماء أخلطت به شيئًا من مائية الدم ومرّة صفراء . أولى البحران .

٥ . أحمد أصناف البول ما كان حسن اللون فيه غمامة بيضاء ملساء مستوية . إمّا راسبة في أسفل القارورة وهو الأفضل . أو متعلّقة في الوسط وهو دون الأوّل أو طافية من فوق وهو دون الثاني . فهذه الثلاثة أصناف هي التي تدلّ على النضج . فأمّا جميع أصناف البول الباقية فبعضها يدلّ على خلاف النضج وبعضها يدلّ على التلف . أولى البحران .

٦ . الاستواء المشترط به في الرسوب ضربان . أحدهما أن لا يكون متفرّقا متشتّتا بل مجتمع والثاني أن يكون كذلك في جميع الأوقات . لأنّه قد تجد البول صافيا في وقت وفيه رسوب في وقت آخر ولا يستمرّ ظهور الرسوب المحمود . وذلك دليل على أنّ النضج لم يستكمل . أولى البحران .

٧ . أجود أبوال المرضى هو الذي يظهر فيه عند خروجه الرسوب المحمود الكامل الصفات . فإنّه يدلّ على أنّ الطبيعة قد ظهرت على المرض وأخذت في إخراج الخلط الممرّض . وبعده في الجودة الذي يبال كدرا وبعد خروجه بقليل يرسب فيه

---

٢ للمرض] للمريض S || ١٥ يستمرّ] يستتمّ B

for this indicates that nature has begun its work and will soon complete it. The third-best urine is that which is turbid when it is excreted but then becomes clear, with no sediment deposited in it, [for] this indicates that the time of the coction is [still] far away, although nature has begun to desire it. *De crisibus* 1.[14]

(8) Someone who is afflicted by fever because of ease of life, rest, and overeating unavoidably deposits much sediment in [his] urine. But as for those who are afflicted by fever because of taking a small amount [of food][15] and because of exertion, their illness often terminates without anything settling in their urine. A sufficient indication for coction is the appearance of a white, smooth, even cloud on top of the urine or suspended in its middle. *De crisibus* 1.[16]

(9) When diseases originate from crude humors, there is much sediment in the urine. When they originate from bilious humors, there is no sediment at all or only a small amount. *In Hippocratis Prognostica commentarius* 2.[17]

(10) The worst urine for ill people is the one that is thin and clear, that truly[18] resembles water and persists in that [resemblance], and is as far as possible from being cocted. Second in bad quality is the urine which is thin and clear when it is excreted but then becomes turbid after a short time, for this indicates that nature, although it has not [yet] started its work, will soon do so. Third in bad quality is the urine which is excreted turbid and stays like that, for this indicates that nature has begun to desire the coction but has not yet [processed] anything. *De crisibus* 1.[19]

(11) Among the kidney ailments is one in which the patient urinates thin, watery fluid similar to the excrement discharged in the beginning of a liver affection. This [discharge] is a bit more like blood than [that] first mentioned. *De locis affectis* 6.[20]

رسوب محمود . فإنّه يدلّ على أنّ الطبيعة قد أخذت في العمل وعن قريب يكمل عملها . ودون هذا الثاني في الجودة الذي يبال كدرا ثمّ يصفو ولا يرسب فيه رسوب . فإنّه يدلّ أنّ وقت الإنضاج بعيد وإن كانت الطبيعة قد بدأت ترومه . أولى البحران .

٨ . يرسب ضرورة في بول من يعتريه الحمّى من الخفض والدعة والإكثار من الطعام رسوبا كثيرا . وأمّا الذين يعتريهم الحمّى من الإقلال والتعب فكثيرا ما ينقضي مرضهم من غير أن يرسب شيء في أبوالهم . وتكتفي في الاستدلال على النضج بظهور غمامة بيضاء ملساء مستوية في أعلى الماء أو متعلّقة في وسطه . أولى البحران .

٩ . إذا حدثت الأمراض عن أخلاط نيئة كان الرسوب في البول كثيرا . وإذا كان حدوثها عن أخلاط صفراوية فلا يكون رسوب أصلا أو يكون قليلا . في شرحه لثانية تقدمة المعرفة .

١٠ . شرّ أبوال المرضى كلّها هو الرقيق الصافي الشبيه بالماء على الصحّة والاستقصاء الباقي كذلك وهو في الغاية القصوى من البعد عن النضج . ودونه في الشرّ الذي يبال رقيقا صافيا وبعد خروجه بقليل ينكدر فإنّه يدلّ على أنّ الطبيعة وإن كانت لم تأخذ في العمل فعن قريب تعمل . ودون هذا الثاني في الشرّ الذي يبال كدرا ويبقى كدرا فإنّه يدلّ على أنّ الطبيعة قد بدأت تروم النضج ولم تميّز بعد شيئا . أولى البحران .

١١ . من علل الكليتين علّة يبول فيها صاحبها صديدا رقيقا شبيها بالبراز الذي يخرج في ابتداء علّة الكبد . وهذا أكثر دموية من ذلك قليلا . سادسة التعرّف .

---

٤ الخفض] الخفظ S || ٨ نيئة] فجّة L

(12) If the diarrhea[21] is of the type of the bilious humor and is oily, it indicates the melting of the fat through the heat of the fever. If the urine is oily and its color and consistency are like the color and consistency of olive oil, it is an indication of death, because it comes from the melting of the flesh; for the heat which melts the flesh is stronger than the heat which melts the fat. *In Hippocratis Epidemiarum* 3.3.[22]

(13) When urine resembling water is micturated quickly, it is the disease called diabetes. This urine is the worst of the uncocted urines; and it [indicates], as it were, the death of two of the natural faculties—namely, the alterative and retentive faculties. *De crisibus* 1.[23]

(14) A black sediment indicates either fiery heat or extreme cold, which result in a condition similar to the death of the natural faculties. A lead-colored[24] [sediment] originates from cold alone. *De crisibus* 1.[25]

(15) Any urine that turns black is so extremely malignant that I do not know anyone who has micturated black urine and survived. But a black sediment indicates a less serious threat of death. If there is a black cloud in the middle of the urine, it indicates a less serious threat of death than a black sediment. [And] a black cloud floating [on top of the urine] is a less serious indication of death than that suspended in the middle [of the urine]. *De crisibus* 1.[26]

(16) If urine that is as white and fine as water has a cloud floating on top of it, or if it has a black sediment or what appears to be dark sediment,[27] or if it contains particles similar to cereal[28] or flakes,[29] all of [these] are fatal [signs]. Similarly, urine with a terrible smell and fatty urine which is called oily are both fatal. These urines indicate that the illness is of a very serious nature. *De totius morbi temporibus liber.*[30]

١٢ . إذا كان اختلاف من جنس المرار دســما فذلك دليل على ذوبان الشــحم من حرارة الحمّى . وإذا كان البول دسما ولونه وقوامه كلون الزيت وقوامه فذلك دليل هلاك لأنّه مــن ذوبان اللحم . والحرارة التي تذيب اللحم أقوى من الحرارة التي تذيب الشحم . في الثالثة من شرحه لثالثة ابيديميا .

١٣ . إذا كان خروج البول الشبيه بالماء سريعا وهي العلّة التي تسمّى ذيابيطس . فذلك شــرّ الأبــوال الغير نضجــة وكأنّه موت قوّتين مــن القوى الطبيعيــة : المغيّرة والماسكة . أولى البحران .

١٤ . الرسوب الأسود يدلّ إمّا على حرارة نارية أو على برد مفرط يعرض منه حال شبيه بالموت للقوى الطبيعية . واللون الرصاصي إنّما يتولّد عن البرد فقط . أولى البحران .

١٥ . كلّ بول يصير إلى السواد فهو رديء في غاية الرداءة حتى أنّي لا أعلم أحدا ممّن بال أسود سلم . وأمّا الرسوب الأسود فدلالته على التلف أقلّ . وإن كانت غمامة ســوداء في وســط الماء فهي أقلّ دلالة على التلف من الرسوب الأسود . والغمامة السوداء الطافية أقلّ دلالة على الهلاك من المتعلّقة في الوسط . أولى البحران .

١٦ . البول الأبيض الرقيق مثل الماء إذا كانت في أعلاه غمامة طافية أو رسوب أســود أو رأيته مظلما أو فيه أجزاء شبيهة بالســويق أو بالصفائح فذلك كلّه قتّال . وكذلك البول الشــديد النتن أو الدســم وهو المســمّى الزيتي جميعا مهلكان . وهذه الأبوال تدلّ على أنّ المرض في طبيعته عظيمة . في مقالته في أوقات الأمراض .

---

١٤ طافية] ساكنة ELBP

(17) Any color of the urine apart from white, yellow, and red is a sign of death. Similarly, anything which appears in the urine apart from a sediment or a cloud in a suspended or floating state—all three of which are laudable—is either a bad or a fatal sign. *De crisibus* 1.[31]

(18) If the illness is prolonged and slow to move[32] and the patient passes thin urine for a long time, the crisis usually comes with an abscess. If he passes much urine which is thick and contains a laudable sediment deposited [in it], it is most likely[33] that the illness will coct gradually and that there will not be a crisis with an abscess. *De crisibus* 3.[34]

(19) If [there] appear in the urine white particles similar to particles of bitter vetch[35] or of lentils,[36] it indicates that they come from the liver. If these particles are similar to flesh, it indicates that they come from the kidneys; and, if they are similar to flakes, it indicates that they come from the urinary bladder. Particles [which are] similar to cereal in size and hardness and [are] not white indicate dissolution in the flesh of the organs. Black particles indicate dissolution in the flesh of the spleen. Oily urine indicates dissolution of the fat. Urine similar to that of animals indicates a large amount of crude matter. *In Hippocratis Epidemiarum* 6.5.[37]

(20) Says Moses: Galen's words in *De crisibus* can be summarized [to this effect]: The best urine of ill people is the one in which—when micturated—a laudable sediment is seen. This one is called the first because nature has completed its activity and cocted the illness-producing matter. Second best is the urine which is turbid when it is micturated and becomes clear once it is micturated while a laudable sediment settles in it, for this indicates that nature has started its work and will soon finish it. This is the second[-best] urine. The third-best urine is the one which is turbid when it is micturated and then becomes clear without a sediment settling in it, for this indicates that nature has started its work but has not approached

١٧ . كلّ لـون يكون في البول غير الأبيـض والأصفر والأحمر فهو دليل تلف. وكذلـك كلّمـا يظهر في البول خارجا عن الرسـوب أو الغمامـة المتعلّقة أو الطافية المحمودة ثلاثتها فهو إمّا دليل رديء أو دليل هلاك. أولى البحران.

١٨ . إذا كان المـرض متطاولا بطيء الحركة وبال المريض بولا رقيقا زمانا طويلا فمـن عادة البحران أن يكون فيه بخراج. وإن بال بولا كثيرا ثخينا فيه ثفل راسـب محمود فالأخلق أن ينضج المرض قليلا قليلا ولا يحدث بحران بخراج. ثالثة البحران.

١٩ . إذا خرج في البول قطع شـبيهة بفتات الكرسنّة أو فتات العدس دلّ على أنّها من الكبد. وإن كانت تلك القطع شـبيهة باللحـم دلّت على أنّها من الكلى وإن كانت شبيهة بالصفائح دلّت على أنّها من المثانة. والقطع الشبيهة بالسويق في قدرها وصلابتها وليست بيضاء تدلّ على أنّ الذوبان في لحم الأعصاب. والقطع السود تدلّ على أنّ الذوبان في لحم الطحال. والبول الدسـم يدلّ على ذوبان الشـحم. والشبيه ببول الدوابّ يدلّ على كثرة الخام. في خامسة شرحه لسادسة ابيديميا.

٢٠ . قال موسـى: الذي تلخّص من كلام جالينوس في البحران أنّ أفضل أبوال المرضى الذي يبال وقد ظهر فيه الرسـوب المحمود ويسمّى هذا الأوّل لأنّ الطبيعة قد استكملت فعلها وأنضجت المادّة الممرضة. ويليه في الجودة البول الذي يبال كدرا ثمّ بعد خروجه يصفو ويرسب رسوب محمود فإنّه يدلّ على أنّ الطبيعة قد أخذت في العمل وعن قريب يكمل عملها وهو البول الثاني. ثمّ يليه في الجودة الذي يبال كدرا ثمّ يصفو ولا يرسب فيه رسوب فإنّه يدلّ على أنّ الطبيعة قد أخذت في العمل ولم يقرب

---

١ دليل] يدلّ على S || ١٠–١١ لحم . . . في] om. G

the time of coction. This is the third[-best urine]. The fourth-best urine is the one which is turbid when it is micturated and then stays turbid, for this one is [even] further away from coction than the previous urine. This is the fourth[-best urine]. Next [the fifth-best] is the urine which is micturated clear and thin and then becomes turbid, for this indicates that nature has not yet begun its work but will shortly do so. The worst urine is that which is micturated thin and then remains that way, for this indicates a total absence of coction, both in the present condition and in the near future.

This is the end of the fifth treatise,
by the grace of God, praise be to Him.

وقت الإنضاج وهو الثالث. ويليه في الجودة وهو يبال كدرا ويبقى كدرا فإنّ هذا أبعد عن النضج من الذي قبله وهو الرابع. يليه الذي يبال صافيا رقيقا ثمّ يتكدّر فإنّه يدلّ على أنّ الطبيعة بعد لم تأخذ في العمل لكنّها عن قريب تبدأ أن تعمل. وأردأ الأبوال الذي يبال رقيقا ويبقى على رقّته فإنّ هذا أدلّ على عدم النضج بالكلّية لا في الحالة الحاضرة ولا في ما قرب. تمّت المقالة الخامسة وللّه الحمد والمنّة.

---

٤ أدلّ] om. B يـدلّ EL || ٥ تمّـت المقالة الخامسـة وللّه الحمد والمنّـة] om. B : كملت المقالة الخامسة وعدد فصولها ثمانية عشر فصلا L : كملت المقالة الخامسة وعدد فصولها ثمانية عشر فصلا والحمد للّه ربّ العالمين E : كملت المقالة الخامسة P

Supplement

Critical comparison of the Arabic text with the Hebrew translations and the previous translation into English

1.6: فلذلك متى يمتدّ جنس العصب شاركته العروق الضوارب في الألم ("Therefore, if the nerves are stretched, the arteries share in the pain"); פ translates: ולכן כשימתח בשר העצב משריקה ימצאו בו העורקים הדופקים. Instead of the correct ימתח ("to stretch," for يمتدّ), r reads: ינתח ("to dissect"). Disregarding the corrupt משריקה (for شاركته), he translates: "Thus, if one dissects the fleshy substance of a nerve, one will discover therein the arteriolar endings." ב translates شاركته correctly as: ישתתפו עמו הגידים.

1.7: الرباطات المدوّرة ("the round ligaments"); reading المدوّرة as الممدودة ("stretched"), פ translates: המתוחים, but ב translates correctly: הקשרים העגולים.

1.15: والمحرّك للشفتين والعينين ("and which move the lips and the eyes"); instead of the correct translation המניעים for والمحرّك, פ has a faulty version: המגיעים; r translates this as: "and which surround the lips" (n. 15: literally "reach"). ב has a correct translation: והמניע.

1.18: إمّا أن يحزّ في العظم ("either a groove is made into the bone"); not reading يحزّ (διατιτράμενον) but يحوي, פ translates: יקיף ("surrounds"), which is translated by r as "encircles." ב's version for يحزّ is unclear.

Ibid.: حدبة العظم ("the convexity of the bone"); פ's incorrect translation: תנועת העצם ("the movement of the bone") is based on reading حدبة as حركة. r translates this as: "no movement of bone." ב provides the same translation as פ.

1.21: الأعضاء التي تظنّ بها أنّها في البدن مفردة هي بالحقيقة زوج مثل الدماغ ("Organs [generally] considered unpaired in the body are in reality paired, such as the brain . . ."); based on פ's defective version: האברים שיחשב בהם שהם נפרדים בגוף, באמת הם המוח, which does not translate the Arabic زوج مثل ("paired, such as"), **r** translates: "organs which are considered unpaired in the body are verily the brain . . ." ב translates زوج مثل as: (?)זוגיו.

1.22: وعصب تخصّه ("and specific nerves"); not reading تخصّه but ثخينة, פ translates: עבים. Following פ, **r** translates: "thick nerves." ב translates correctly: ועצב יחדהו.

1.27: وليس فعل العضل فيها حينئذ متعطّل ("and the activity of the muscles is not abolished at that time"); פ's correct translation: ואין פעל העצלים בהם אז בטל is corrupted by **m** as: ואין פעל העצלים בהם, או הבטל. This is the basis for **r**'s translation: "The muscles are not active; they are idle."

1.34: ولا حلّ الشكّ الذي يروم حلّه ("neither did he resolve the doubt—although it calls for a solution"); פ does not read ولا حلّ but ولأجل (cf. variant **E**) and translates: ובשויל הספק אשר נרצה לגלותו. **r** translates this as: "because of the uncertainty which needs clarification." ב translates this as: ולא התיר הספק אשר יחשוב להתירו.

1.35: الحركات الإرادية قد تكون تابعة لفكرة وروية كحركتنا لرصد كوكب من الكواكب ("Voluntary movement sometimes follows from thought and reflexion as in our movement to observe a certain star"); reading وروية كحركتنا as ومقوية حركتنا ("strengthening our movement") and لرصد as لركض ("running"), פ corrupts the Arabic as: התנועה הרצונית לפעמים יהיו נמשכות למחשבה, ומחזק בתנועתינו למרוצת כוכב מהכוכבים. Following פ, **r** translates: "Voluntary movement is sometimes derived from active thought which strengthens our movement to run to the most distant star." ב translates the section وروية كحركتنا لرصد كوكب correctly as: וראיה כתנועתנו לראות כוכב מן הכוכבים.

1.38: هو تابع إمّا لمجرّد الخيال ("result either from imagination only"); not reading لمجرّد الخيال, but لحدث الخيال, פ translates: למחדש הדמיון. **r** translates this as: "active imagination." ב translates this section correctly as: לדמיון פשוט.

1.43: كي يطول مقام الدم هناك ("in order that the blood will stay there for a long time"); reading يطول as يكون, פ translates: כדי שיעמוד מקום הדם, and **r**:

"in order that the blood is slowed sufficiently." ב translates the section correctly as: כדי שיאריך במקום הדם.

1.45: وإنّا يعرض مرارا كثيرة أن ينضرّ حسّ المذاق ("It often happens that the sense of taste is harmed"); the term ينضرّ has a variant in **SG**: يتغيّر. This variant is read by פ as يتعيّن and translated as: שיעויין. **r** translates this as: "is destroyed" (?). ב translates the variant reading of **SG** correctly as: ישתנה, while a marginal gloss provides a correct translation for ينضرّ, namely, ינזק.

1.48: ناتئا عن ("above"); reading this term as تأتي عن, פ translates: יבואה מן, and **r**: "originating from." ב translates this as: יוצא ל- ("outside").

1.54: بزوائدها ("by its lobes"); פ's correct version ביתרותיה is read by **m** as: ביתדותיה and translated by **r** as: "to its supports." ב translates the term correctly as: עם התוספות.

1.55: وأخفّ ("lighter"); reading this term as وأجفّ, פ translates: נגוב, and **r**: "drier." ב has a correct translation: יותר קל.

1.60: حياة ("life"); reading this term as حيوان, פ translates: בעלי חיים, and **r**: "living beings." ב has a translation similar to פ : הבעל חיים.

1.61: لرداءة الخلط الذي يسلك فيه ("Because of the badness of the humor which streams through it"); reading يسلك as يتولد, פ translates: לרוע הליחה אשר תתילד בו, and **r**: "because of the bad quality of the humor which is produced in it." ב translates يسلك correctly as: תלך.

1.67: دون ("unlike"); understanding this term in its literal sense of "beneath," פ translates: יורד למטה and **r**: "descends below." ב translates it correctly as: זולתי.

2.1: الدم هو الشيء المركّب من جميع الأخلاط ("Blood is something composed of all the humors"): **m** has corrupted פ's version הדם הוא דבר מורכב מכל הליחות as: הדם הוא דבר מורכב מעל הליחות, and **r** has translated this as: "Blood is something superior to all humors."

2.3: المرّة الصفراء مشبعة كانت أو غير مشبعة ("The yellow bile, whether it is saturated or not"); **r** regards פ's transcription מצובעת for مشبعة as a Hebrew word derived from צבע ("color") and therefore translates: "The red bile appears either dyed with color or without color."

2.7: دردي (*durdī*: "lees of wine"); פ transcribes this as דורדי, which is read by **m** as: דורדיא and transcribed by **r** as: *durdaya.* ב translates this term correctly as: שמרים ("dregs"). (Cf. 3.61, where both פ and ב have שמרי היין.)

Ibid.: ويشتوي من الحرارة النارية ("is roasted because of the fiery heat"); **m** reads פ's version: ויחרצו(?) מן החום הטבעי as: ויחרגו מן החום הטבעי. This is translated by **r** as: "exceed their natural heat." ב translates the Arabic correctly as ותקלה ("and is roasted").

2.17: الكيموس يقال له الخام ("The chyme which is called 'crude'"); פ's transcription אלכאם is read by **m** as: אלכא"ם and is then transcribed by **r** as "El Quʾam" (cf. "Elqaʾis," 3.45). In 23.3, he transcribes it correctly as *"alcham."* ב translates it as: אלנא בער' אלכם בלעז קרודו ("the crude," in Arabic *al-khām,* in Romance *qrwdw*).

Ibid.: من يحمّ من كثرة النخم ("Someone who suffers from fever due to a surplus of raw phlegms"); פ reads يحسّ for يحمّ and الحمّى for النخم, and thus translates: מי שירגיש מפני רוב הקדחת, which is the basis for **r**: "one who has high fever." ב translates the sentence correctly as: מי שיש לו קדחת מפני ריבוי המילוי הנק' אמפוניטו ("someone who suffers from fever because of an overfilling called '*ʾmpwnyṭw*'").

2.23: وقد تدفع المرارة إلى الكبد بالعنق بعينها التي جذبت بها ("Sometimes the bile is expelled towards the liver through the neck [of the gallbladder] itself, by which it is attracted"): פ reading بعينها ("itself") as بينهما, ("between them") translates: ביניהם ("between them"); accordingly **r** translates: "Sometimes the bile finds its way to the liver through the neck which is between them through which secretions pour." ב does not translate the Arabic بعينها.

2.25: الورم الساعي ("shingles"); פ translates: והמורסא המתחברת while ב provides a more correct translation: והמורסא השורצת כלו המתפשטת הנה והנה.

3.4: بدن الرجال كلّه يتنفّس تنفّسا جيّدا وهو نقي معرّى من الفضول ("The whole body of a man breathes well when it is clean and free of superfluities"); פ's translation for وهو نقي معرّى من الفضول, namely, והוא נקי תמנע מהמותרים, is corrupted by **m** as: והוא נקי מהאצטומכא תמנע מהמותרים. This is the basis for **r**'s corruption: "Metabolism in man's body proceeds well, providing the stomach is clean and free of superfluities."

3.5: خير عظيم لهم ليس بيسير الموقع ("is of great benefit to them and provides quite a few opportunities"); פ's version: אינה מטובות הטוב is read by **m** as: אינה מעכבת הטוב. The term מטובות in פ has been corrected in the margin as: מעוטת(?).

3.13: الأشياء الملينة المسكّة ("Ingredients which soften, alleviate..."); disregarding الملينة and reading المسخنة instead of المسكّة, פ translates: הדברים המחממים, and **r**: "warming substances." ב does translate الملينة correctly as: הדברים המחליקים but gives the same translation as פ for المسكّة.

3.18: وطلوع السماك هو أوّل الخريف ("The rising of Virgo is the beginning of autumn"); transcribing السماك as אל סימאך, פ translates: ועלית אלסמאך הוא תחלת החורף. **m** interprets אל סימאך as a plural from سمكة ("fish") and thus explains the term as הדגים ("fishes"). Accordingly **r** translates: "The rising of the constellation of *Al-Semach,* referring to fish, ushers in the beginning of autumn." ב gives the same transcription as פ.

3.19: صالحة في العظم وفي العدد ("[veins] which were quite important and numerous"); not reading عظم as *ᶜizam* ("importance"), but as *ᶜazm* ("bone"), and not reading عدد ("number"), but غدد ("gland"), פ translates: נכונים בעצם ובגדרים. Accordingly, **r** translates: "good veins reformed in bone or in glands." ב translates like פ: הרבה בעצמות ובגרנדולי ("many [veins] in the bones and glands"). (Romance *gr'ndwly* means glands.)

3.34: في جرم الكبد ("In the body of the liver"); פ translates جرم correctly as: גרם ("body"). **m** corrupts this as: הדם ("the blood"), and following **m**, **r** translates: "in the blood of the liver."

3.42: والنفخة التي لا قرعة معها ("exsufflation without noise"); פ's correct translation for قرعة, namely, הלימה, is corrupted by **m** as: הליחה ("sputum"). **r** accordingly translates: "cough unassociated with sputum."

Ibid.: ومتى نال الفعل الواحد من هذه الخمسة مضرّة إنضرّ كلّما بعده ولا ينضرّ ما قبله ("When one of these functions is damaged, all the following ones are damaged [as well], but not the previous ones"); פ, reading إنضرّ as انظر ("look") and ينضرّ as ينظر ("to look"), translates the last part of the sentence as: עיין אל מה שאחריו ואל תביט אל מה שלפניו ("look at what is after it, but not at what is before it"). This is the basis for **r**: "Should any one of these five functions be damaged, one should take heed of the next one and not look at the previous one." ב translates the second part correctly as: ינזק כל שאר אחריו ולא ינזק כל מה שלפניו ("all the ones that come after it are damaged, but not the ones before it").

3.49: حرارة مكتسبة ("acquired heat"); פ translates this term correctly as חום קנוי. However, **m** misinterprets פ's translation as חום קרוי. This is the basis for **r**'s translation: "accidental heat."

3.54: العصبة التي تنبثّ وتتفرّق في العضلة ("the nerve that spreads in the muscle"); not reading تنبثّ ("to spread") but تنبت ("to grow"), פ translates: כי העצב אשר צומח ומתפזר בעצל. **r** translates this as: "the nerve that grows and divides within that muscle." ב's version is similar to that of פ.

3.58: ربّما سكن البدن السكون والدعة ("Sometimes the body is at rest and ease"); not reading سكن but سخن , פ translates: לפעמים יתחמם הגוף בהשקט ומנוחה, which **r** translates as: "Sometimes . . . it is afflicted with high temperature." ב translates: אפשר שתצוה לעשות לגוף מנוחה ונחת ("Sometimes one is ordered to rest and relax the body").

3.59: وهذا الجنس من العفونة ليس هو عفونة فقط بل يشوبه نضج ("This kind of putrefaction is not merely putrefaction but is mixed with coction"); not reading يشوبه but يشبه, פ translates: וזה המין מהעפוש איננו עפוש אבל דומה [ל]בשול. This is translated by **r** as: "This type of putrefaction is not true decay but rather a form of digestion." ב provides a correct translation of the Arabic: וזה הסוג מן העיפוש אינו הוא עיפוש לבדו אבל יתערב עמו בישול.

3.61: الدبيلات ("abscesses"); correctly translated and transcribed by פ as: מורסות הנקראות דבילות; **m** corrupts it as: המורסות הנקראות רמלות (cf. n. 81); and **r** translates this as: "abscesses which are called 'groat-bags.'" ב has a version similar to פ: מורסות הנקראות דבילות.

3.63: عفن ذلك الدم كما تعفن أبدان الموتى وإن كانت باقية ولم تخرج خروجا كثيرا قويت على ذلك الدم وأحالته مدّة (". . . that blood putrefies just as the bodies of the dead putrefy. But if the innate heat remains [in a balanced state] and does not deviate too much from it, it prevails over that blood and transforms it into pus"); פ translates وإن كانت باقية as: ואע"פ שהם נשארים קדומים, whereby the number of the predicate does not correspond to the subject ("blood") but to the preceding word ("bodies"). פ's version קדומים is misread by **m** as: קרומים. This is the basis for **r**'s translation: "Even if they remain covered with membranes." It is clear that **r** did not recognize the phenomenon typical for medieval Hebrew translations from the Arabic that required the number of the predicate to correspond to the preceding word (see Bos, *Aristotle's* De anima, 24–25).

3.64: ويرتفع الإحساس بالألم ("and the sensation of pain stops"); פ's corrupt translation: ויגבהו וינפחו הגשמים ויחוש בכאב seems to have been caused by reading the Arabic as: ويرتفع وينتفخ الأجسام ويحسّ بالألم . Following פ (edition **m**), **r** translates: "If a swelling or distention occurs, pain is felt (again)." ב translates this section correctly as: והכאב יסור מעליו.

3.86: وكل الأمر كلّه حينئذ إلى الطبيعة ("In this case the whole matter should be left to nature"); not reading وكل (*wakil* = "and entrust") but وأصل ("and the root"), פ translates: ושורש זה הענין כלו הוא אל הטבעי. **r** translates this as: "The fundamental principle under these conditions is that everything should be left to nature." ב translates وكل correctly as: והניח.

3.88: لا يكاد يكون في الصدر والكبد ورم بلغمي ("A phlegmatic tumor hardly ever occurs in the chest and liver"); פ, reading لا يكاد يكون as لا تظنّ أن يكون, translates it as: לא תחשוב שיהיה בכבד and بلغمي as לבניית; following פ, **r** translates: "Do not think that a white abscess can occur in the liver or chest." ב translates لا يكاد يكون as: אי אפשר להיות ("it is impossible that"), and for بلغمي he provides the Romance equivalent: פליאומטיקא (*phly'wmṭyq'*).

3.93: وهو صرف بحدته دائما ("It [i.e., the jejunum] is the only [organ] that is always free [of food]"); reading صرف ("pure") as صدف ("to encounter," form III) and deriving حدته from حرّ ("heat") and not from وحد ("to be unique"), פ translates: והוא פוגע בחומה תמיד. **r**, deriving בחומה from חומה ("wall") and not from חום ("heat"), translates: "It is also constantly touching the (intestinal) wall." ב does not translate this section.

3.105: ولا تدرّ البول إن ابتدأ حدوث ورم في المثانة والإحليل والكليتين ("And do not prescribe diuretics when a tumor begins to appear in the urinary bladder, penis, or kidneys."); פ, reading دم instead of ورم, translates إن ابتدأ حدوث ورم في المثانة as: כשיתחיל התחדשות דם המקוה ("when bleeding of the urinary bladder occurs"), and **r**, following פ, translates: "Also do not give diuretics when bleeding occurs from the urinary bladder or urethra or both kidneys." ב translates this part correctly as: אם התחילה המורסא בשלפוחית ("When a tumor appears in the urinary bladder").

Ibid.: فلا تحدر الحيض في ابتداء حدوث ورم في الرحم أو الفرج ("And do not induce menstruation when a tumor first appears in the uterus or vulva"); פ, reading الفرج as القرح, translates this as: אבעבועות ("boils"), and **r** translates פ as: "Similarly, do not induce menstruation at the beginning of a uterine abscess or blister formation." ב translates أو الفرج correctly as: או בערוה ("or in the vulva").

3.107: إذا علّقت المحجمة على القفاء في موضع الفأس كانت من أقوى الأشياء نفعا في منع انصباب المواد إلى العين ("When one applies cupping glasses to the neck on the occipital protuberance, it is one of the best means to prevent the [superfluous] matters from streaming towards the eye"); פ corrupts في موضع الفأس as: העצם הנקרא הקרדוס and translates: כשתתלה קרן המציצה על העורק במקום העצם הנקרא הקרדוס. **r** translates this as: "If one applies a suction cup on the vessel over the site of the bone called *hekardos*." ב corrupts الفأس as החפירה.

4.2: فإنّ لهذين الزمانين أحدهما عند الآخر بلا شكّ نسبة ما طبيعية بحسب كلّ واحد من الأسنان ("The proportion between these two times is 'without any doubt' according to what is natural for each of the [different] ages [of man]"); reading اثنان ("two") instead of أسنان ("ages"), פ translates: כי אלו ב' הזמנים אחד מהם אצל האחר בלי ספק יש יחס מהטבעי כפי כל אחד מהשניים. **r** translates: "These two times are complementary to each other." ב translates بحسب كلّ واحد من الأسنان as: וישתנה ולפעמים ישתנה.

4.9: أو الآفة الحادثة بالآلة ("or from an affliction occurring to the organ"); פ translates: או הפגע המתחדש, omitting بالآلة ("to the organ"). **m** emends the deficient text of פ with באצטומכה ("in the stomach"), which is the basis for **r**: "or due to an affliction arising in the stomach." ב has the complete version: או החלי המתחדש בכלי.

4.14: النبض الخامل ("the faint pulse"); reading الخامل as الكامل, פ translates: הדפק השלם. **r** translates this as: "a normal pulse." ב is identical to פ.

4.15: يوهم أنّ جرم العرق قد تفتّت ("It seems as if the body of the artery has fragmented"); פ's correct translation of تفتّت, namely, נתפתת, is corrupted by **m** as נתפתח; hence **r**'s translation: "which appears and is thought of as being due to holes in the artery."

4.16: ولا تكاد تجد ("one hardly ever finds"); not reading تكاد but تظنّ (?), פ translates: ולא יחשוב שימצא. This is translated by **r** as: "and therefore (one should) be unconcerned if one finds." ב translates the Arabic as: ולא תוכל למצוא ("One cannot find").

4.23: أو عريا عن الصلابة ("but not hard"); not reading عريا عن ("without"), but عن ("from, of"), פ translates: או מן הקשי. This is translated by **r** as: "or hard." ב has a correct translation: או ערום מן הקושי.

4.26: لكنّ هناك مادّة كثيرة قد ثقلت على القوة ("but it is burdened . . . by a large amount of [superfluous] matter"); perhaps reading نقلت ("to transport") instead of ثقلت, פ translates: אך שיש שם ליחה רבה שנשפכה על הכח. **r** translates this as: "except if an excess of humor pours over it." ב translates the sentence correctly as: אבל יש שם חומר מרובה שיכבד על הכח.

4.33: كما يعقب النبض الموجي . . . النبض الدودي ("As the undulatory pulse . . . is followed by the vermicular one, so the vermicular pulse . . . is followed by the antlike pulse"); wrongly considering النبض الموجي as the subject and النبض الدودي as the object, פ translates: כמו שמשאיר אחריו הדפק הגלי... הדפק התולעי. This is translated by **r** as: "Just as a fluttering pulse leaves behind a vermiculate pulse." ב translates this section correctly as: כמו שהדפק הגלי... יבוא אחריו הדפק התולעי. The same mistake is repeated in the second part of the paragraph.

4.40: إلا إن ينضاف إلى ذلك أحد الثلاثة الأسباب ("when it is joined by one of the three [other] causes"); פ translates: אלא אם יצטרך לזה אחת מג' סבות. The term יצטרך ("to need") for ينضاف ("to add") is possibly a scribal error for יצטרף. **r** translates this as: "except in one of the three situations." ב translates this term correctly as: יחובר.

4.41: يبلّ ("moistens"); deriving يبلّ from بلا ("to test," form VIII: "to suffer"), פ translates: סובל, which might be a scribal error for טובל. **r** (n. 62) translates it as "burden." ב has the correct version: יטבול.

4.48: متفتّتا ("crumbled"); פ's correct translation מתפתת has been corrupted by **m** as: מתוכיי and corrected as: נמוך; hence **r**'s translation: "low."

5.1: إذ لا تنفكّ ذات الجنب عن حمّى ("because pleuritis does not occur without fever"); פ probably transcribes an Arabic variant for تنفكّ, namely, تخلى ("to be free from") as תכלא. **r** translates this incorrectly as: "because pleuritis is not ordinarily one of the fever-producing illnesses." ב translates تنفكّ عن correctly as: נמלט מ-.

5.8: الإقلال <من الطعام> (“to take a small amount [of food]”); פ derives الإقلال from the root كلّ (“to be tired”) and thus translates: היגיעה. Accordingly, **r** translates: “work.” ב has the same translation as פ.

Ibid.: وتكتفي في الاستدلال على النضج بظهور غمامة بيضاء ملساء مستوية في أعلى الماء (“A sufficient indication for coction is the appearance of a white, smooth, even cloud on top of the urine”); פ, reading وتكتفي as وتختفي, translates this term as: ויסתם (“and is concealed”). פ’s translation of في الاستدلال, namely, מהורות, is corrupted by **m** as במהירות (“hastily”). This results in **r**’s translation: “They rapidly complete the cooking with the appearance of a white, flat, and even turbidity in the upper part of the urine.” ב provides a correct translation of وتكتفي في الاستدلال على النضج as: ויספיק הסימן על הבישול (“to indicate coction it is sufficient”).

5.10: على الصحّة (“truly”); פ’s correct translation באמת is corrupted by **m** as: של בארות and is translated by **r** as: “well [water].”

Ibid.: وإن كانت لم تأخذ في العمل (“although it has not [yet] started its work”); reading تأخذ as تأخّر, פ translates: אע״פ שיש לו אחור. **r** translates this as: “although behind in its task.” ב translates correctly: אע״פ שלא התחיל לעשות.

5.11: صديدا (“pus”); deriving صديدا from the root صدىء (“to be rusty”) instead of from صدّ, פ translates it as: חלודה; hence **r**’s translation: “rusty.” ב translates the term correctly as: מוגלא.

5.18: فالأخلق أن ينضج المرض قليلا قليلا (“it is most likely that the illness will coct gradually”); פ translates الأخلق faultily as: התחיל (“to begin”). Accordingly, **r** translates: “and begin to slowly coct the illness.” ב translates this term correctly as: היותר טוב ש-.

Notes to the English Text

Translator's Introduction

Unless otherwise indicated, all translations of quotations in the introduction and notes are my own.

1. For Maimonides' biographical data, see *EI*[2] 3:876–78, s.v. "Ibn Maymūn" (Vajda); *EJ* 11: cols. 754–64, s.v. "Maimonides, Moses" (Rabinowitz); Lewis, "Maimonides, Lionheart and Saladin," 70–75; Goitein, "Ḥayye ha-Rambam," 29–42; Goitein, "Man of Action," 155–67; Maimonides, *Igrot ha-Rambam,* ed. Shailat, 1:19–21; Cohen, "Maimonides' Egypt," 21–34; Ben-Sasson, "Maimonides in Egypt," 3–30; Levinger, "Was Maimonides 'Rais al-Yahud'?" 83–93; Davidson, "Maimonides' Putative Position," 115–28; Kraemer, "The Life of Moses ben Maimon," 413–28. For Maimonides' training as a physician, see Maimonides, *On Asthma,* ed. Bos, xxv–xxx.

2. While his date of birth is traditionally set at 1135, Maimonides himself states in the colophon to his *Commentary on the Mishnah,* completed in 1168, that he was thirty years old and living in Egypt. Goitein, "Man of Action," 155, argues on the basis of this that the actual year of his birth should be put at 1138; see also Leibowitz, "Der Mann und sein Werk," 75–76.

3. According to Graetz, *Geschichte der Juden,* 7:265, it is generally assumed that the family left Córdoba in the year 1148, when the city was conquered by the Almohads. If this is so, and if the year of his birth was indeed 1138, Maimonides would have been ten years old at the time.

4. Goitein, "Man of Action," 163, has shown that Maimonides was already involved in this trade before his younger brother David perished in a shipwreck in 1169 and that he was still engaged in it in 1191, even while practicing medicine. Goitein dates the tragedy to the year 1178 without substantiation, but in Maimonides, *Igrot ha-Rambam,* ed. Shailat, 1:20, it is said to have occurred during 1177–78.

5. See *EI*[2] 4:376–77, s.v. "al-Ḳāḍī al-Fāḍil" (Brockelmann-[Cl. Cahen]).

6. See Davidson, "Maimonides' Putative Position," esp. 127–28.

7. For descriptions of his medical works, see Meyerhof, "Medical Work"; Friedenwald, *The Jews and Medicine,* 1:200–216; Baron, *Philosophy and Science,*

259–62; Ullmann, *Medizin im Islam,* 167–69; *EJ* 11: cols. 777–79, s.v. "[Maimonides, Moses], as Physician" (Muntner); Maimonides, *Shivḥe ha-Rambam,* ed. Avishur, 33–36; Ackermann, "Ärztliche Tätigkeit," 45–46. For a survey of editors and translators of Maimonides' medical works, see Dienstag, "Translators and Editors," 95–135, esp. 116–21 for Muntner's activity.

8. An edition of Moses ibn Tibbon's Hebrew translation appears in Maimonides, *Perush le-firḳe Abuḳrat,* ed. Muntner. For an English translation, see Maimonides' *Commentary on the Aphorisms of Hippocrates,* ed. and trans. Rosner.

9. An edition of Moses ibn Tibbon's Hebrew translation appears in Maimonides, *Same ha-maṿet,* ed. Muntner. For a German translation, see Maimonides, "Gifte und ihre Heilung," trans. Steinschneider, 62–120. A French translation, Maimonides, *Traité des poisons,* trans. Rabbinowicz, was made from the Hebrew but in consultation with the Arabic text. English translations include Maimonides, *Treatise on Poisons and Their Antidotes,* ed. and trans. Muntner, with a facsimile of the Judaeo-Arabic text, MS Paris 1211, and Maimonides, *Poisons, Hemorrhoids, Cohabitation,* ed. and trans. Rosner.

10. Maimonides, *Art of Cure,* trans. and ed. Barzel. The chronology of these major works has not been researched so far and is the object of much dissension and many unfounded conjectures. In my opinion, it should be dealt with once critical editions of these works are available to provide all the relevant data.

11. The Arabic text of the longer version—which is spurious, according to some scholars—has been edited and translated into German by Hermann Kroner and published as "Shʾnēy maʾamarēi ha-Mishgal"; the same publication comprises the edition of two Hebrew translations of the shorter version. The Arabic original of the shorter version has been edited by Kroner with a German translation in "Eine medizinische Maimonides-Handschrift." See also "Maimonides' Treatise to a Prince," ed. and trans. Stern. For English translations of both versions, see Maimonides, *On Sexual Intercourse,* ed. and trans. Gorlin. The short version was also translated in Maimonides, *Poisons, Hemorrhoids, Cohabitation,* ed. and trans. Rosner.

12. For an Arabic edition with German translation, see Kroner, ed. and trans., "Gesundheitsanleitung des Maimonides"; or see it reprinted in *Beiträge zur Geschichte der arabisch-islamischen Medizin:* Aufsätze, ed. Sezgin et al. For an edition of Moses ibn Tibbon's Hebrew translation, see Maimonides, *Hanhagat ha-beriʾut,* ed. Muntner. For an English translation from the Arabic, see *Maimonides' Regimen of Health,* ed. and trans. Bar-Sela, Hoff, and Faris. Translations from the Hebrew include, in German, Maimonides, *Regimen Sanitatis,* ed. Muntner; in English, *Maimonides' Three Treatises on Health,* ed. and trans. Rosner; and in Spanish, Maimonides, *El régimen de salud,* ed. and trans. Ferre. The scholars generally agree that it was composed in 1198. See Leibowitz, "Verschiedene Arten der Weisheit II," 47 (1190 is a typographical error; in the English edition of this issue of the journal *[Ariel],* p. 37, Leibowitz remarks that Maimonides served the sultan from 1198 on); Maimonides, *Sharḥ asmāʾ al-ʿuqqār,* ed. Meyerhof, lvi; and Rosner, in his works "Medical Writings," 2185–90; *Sex Ethics,* 45; and *Treatise on Asthma,* ed. and trans. Rosner, 12.

13. According to Maimonides, *Sharḥ asmāʾ al-ʿuqqār,* ed. Meyerhof, lvi, it was composed around 1200. For an edition of the Arabic text, a medieval Hebrew translation, and a translation into German, see Maimonides, "Der medizinische Schwanengesang des Maimonides," ed. Kroner. Kroner's Arabic text was published again with medieval Latin translations, a facsimile edition of a Hebrew translation, and an English translation in *Maimonides on the Causes of Symptoms,* ed. Leibowitz and Marcus. For an English translation from the Arabic, see *Maimonides' Regimen of Health,* ed. and trans. Bar-Sela, Hoff, and Faris, 32–40; for a German translation, see Maimonides, *Regimen Sanitatis,* ed. Muntner. A new English translation based on previous editions is Maimonides, *Hemorrhoids, Medical Answers,* ed. and trans. Rosner and Muntner.

14. For an Arabic edition with French translation, see Maimonides, *Sharḥ asmāʾ al-ʿuqqār,* ed. Meyerhof; for a Hebrew translation, see Maimonides, *Beʾur shemot refuʾiyot,* ed. Muntner; for an English translation based on Meyerhof, see Maimonides, *Drug Names,* ed. and trans. Rosner.

15. For an edition of the Arabic text, medieval Hebrew translation, and German translation, see Maimonides, "Die Haemorrhoiden," ed. and trans. Kroner. For English translations from the Hebrew, see Maimonides, *Hemorrhoids, Medical Answers,* ed. and trans. Rosner and Muntner, and Maimonides, *Poisons, Hemorrhoids, Cohabitation,* ed. and trans. Rosner.

16. See Maimonides, *On Asthma,* ed. Bos.

17. According to Ullmann, *Medizin im Islam,* 167–68, it was probably composed between 1187 and 1190.

18. Maimonides, *Commentary on the Aphorisms of Hippocrates,* 2.33 (ed. and trans. Schliwski), XXXIII: "Es sprach Hippokrates: Geistige Gesundheit ist bei jeder Krankheit ein gutes Zeichen, ebenso guter Appetit. Das Gegenteil dessen ist ein schlechtes Zeichen." (Hippocrates said: Mental health is a good sign in any disease; likewise a healthy appetite. The opposite of these is a bad sign.) "Es spricht der Kommentator: Das ist klar. Ich habe den Grund dafür in den *Aphorismen,* die ich verfaßt habe, erklärt." (The commentator says: This is clear. I have explained the reason for this in the *Aphorisms* that I composed); cf. *Medical Aphorisms* 6.94 (ed. Bos).

19. Maimonides, *On Asthma* 13.19 (ed. Bos, 90–91).

20. See p. xxix, where MS Gotha 1937 (**G**) is described in detail.

21. According to Meyerhof, "Medical Work," 276, it was composed during the last ten years of his life; Leibowitz, "Maimonides' Aphorisms," 1, remarks that it was rewritten at the end of his life.

22. See Lieber, "Maimonides, the Medical Humanist," 51.

23. Kahle, "Aphorismum Praefatio et Excerpta."

24. Schacht and Meyerhof, "Maimonides against Galen," 53–88 [Arabic section].

25. See Kafaḥ, ed., *Igrot,* 148–67. Kafaḥ transcribed the original Arabic text from **G** into Judaeo-Arabic. The enumeration of the chapters is according to the Hebrew edition prepared by Muntner.

26. Nathan ha-Meʾati's translation was edited for the first time in Lemberg in 1834 and reprinted in Vilna in 1888. A new edition appears in Maimonides,

Pirḳe Mosheh, ed. Muntner. For Nathan ha-Meʾati (of Cento), see Vogelstein and Rieger, *Geschichte der Juden in Rom,* 1:398–400; Steinschneider, *Die hebräischen Übersetzungen,* 766. For the manuscripts of this translation, see Richler, "Manuscripts of Pirke Moshe."

27. *Medical Aphorisms of Moses Maimonides,* ed. and trans. Rosner and Muntner, and its revision, *Aphorisms,* trans. Rosner.

28. On Zeraḥyah, see Vogelstein and Rieger, *Geschichte der Juden in Rom,* 1:271–75, 409–18; Steinschneider, *Die hebräischen Übersetzungen,* 766; Ravitzky, *Mishnato shel R. Zeraḥyah,* 69–75; Bos, *Aristotle's* De Anima, chapter 7: "Zeraḥyah's Technique of Translation." For the manuscripts of this translation, see Richler, "Manuscripts of *Pirke Moshe,*" 352–54. For a list of editions, translations, and studies of the *Medical Aphorisms,* see Dienstag, "Bibliography," 455–70.

29. See Schacht and Meyerhof, "Maimonides against Galen," 59–60. For a general introduction to the *Medical Aphorisms,* see Maimonides, *Pirḳe Mosheh,* ed. Muntner, xii–xviii; Rosner, "Medical Aphorisms of Maimonides," 6–30; *Aphorisms,* trans. Rosner, xii–xxvi; Schacht and Meyerhof, "Maimonides against Galen," 58–63; Bos, "The Reception of Galen in *Medical Aphorisms,*" 139–52.

30. See Maimonides, *Medical Aphorisms* 7.71 (ed. Bos). The numbering of the sections of the different treatises is according to Maimonides, *Pirḳe Mosheh,* ed. Muntner, and *Aphorisms,* trans. Rosner.

31. See Larrain, "Galen, *De motibus dubiis.*"

32. Ibn Abī Uṣaybiʿa, *ʿUyūn al-anbāʾ fī ṭabaqāt al-aṭibbāʾ,* 149; compare Meyerhof, "Schriften Galens," 542 (484), no. 56; Ullmann, "Zwei spätantike Kommentare," 245–62.

33. See 3.76 of translated text, p. 52.

34. See Galen, *De libris propriis* (ed. Kühn, 19:8–48); Bergsträsser, ed. and trans., *Ḥunain ibn Isḥāq;* Bergsträsser, *Ibn Isḥāq's Galen-Bibliographie,* 274–87.

35. See Bos, "A Recovered Fragment," 189–94.

36. See 1.3 of translated text and nn. 6–9 to the first treatise, below; compare Galen, *De usu partium* 9.5 (ed. Helmreich, 2:15–18; trans. May, 1:434–36.)

37. Trans. May, 1:434 n. 14.

38. Quoted in translation by Langermann, "Synochous Fever," 177. Steinschneider, *Die hebräischen Übersetzungen,* 765–66, adducing the introduction, already takes issue with Leclerc's remark that the aphorisms are literal quotations.

39. MS. Wellcome Or. 14a.

40. MS. Gotha 1937 (**G**).

41. The sections in italics in MS Paris 2853 are the ones omitted by Maimonides.

42. Galen, *De sanitate tuenda* 1.5–6 (ed. Koch, 179 lines 12–17); the translation quoted here is from trans. Green, 250. The section in italics has been added by Maimonides.

43. Galen, *De usu partium* 5.5 (ed. Helmreich, 1:266; trans. May, 1:256 n. 20).

44. Schacht and Meyerhof, "Maimonides against Galen," 60.

45. For instance, *Medical Aphorisms* 13.52, 54, 20.83–89, and 22.57–70 (ed. Bos) contain quotations from al-Tamīmī's *Kitāb al-murshid,* which has only been partly preserved; see Ullmann, *Medizin im Islam,* 269–70.

46. See Lieber, "Medical Works of Maimonides: A Reappraisal," 20; as Lieber notes, source references can also be found in al-Rāzī's aphorisms.

47. See Leibowitz, "Latin Translations," XCIII–XCIX, Hebrew version, 273–81; and Dienstag, "Bibliography," 455–57.

48. Maimonides, *Pirḳe Mosheh,* ed. Muntner, xiii.

49. See, for instance, 2.1 of the translated text, p. 26.

50. Cf. Richler, "Manuscripts of *Pirke Moshe,*" 345–47.

51. See Richler, "Another Letter?" 450–52; Shatzmiller, *Jews, Medicine, and Medieval Society,* 46.

52. Ibn Falaquera, *Moreh ha-moreh,* 275–76, ed. Shiffman.

53. For this stone, the name of which is a transcription of Arabic *marqāshīthā,* see Wiedemann, *Aufsätze zur arabischen Wissenschafts-geschichte,* 1:714–16. The text from which Maimonides is quoting—namely, Galen, *Ad Glauconem de methodo medendi* 2.6 (ed. Kühn, 11:107)—does not read "marcasite stone," but "pyrite stone."

54. Maimonides, *Pirḳe Mosheh,* ed. Muntner, xxii, 17 (269–70); *Aphorisms,* trans. Rosner, 343. Galen's text (*Ad Glauconem de methodo medendi* 2.6 [ed. Kühn, 11:107]) reads ἐπὶ δὲ τῶν τενόντων, ὀνομάζω δ' οὕτω δηλονότι τὰς ἀπονευρώσεις τῶν μυῶν, ἐπὶ τῇ λεγομένῃ χρήσει τῶν φαρμάκων ἐναργεστάτην ὠφέλειάν ἐστιν ἰδεῖν, εἴ τις καλῶς χρήσαιτο τῇ διὰ τοῦ πυρίτου λίθου θεραπείᾳ· χρὴ δὲ διάπυρον αὐτὸν ἐργασάμενον ὄξει δριμυτάτῳ καταρραίνειν, εἶτα διακινεῖν τὸ πεπονθὸς μόριον ὑπὲρ τὸν λίθον, ὡς ἂν ὑπὸ τῆς ἀναφερομένης ἀτμίδος ὁ σκίρρος λύοιτο. πολλὰ γὰρ ἤδη τελέως ἠγκυλωμένα τε καὶ κεκυλλωμένα διὰ τούτου τοῦ τρόπου τῆς θεραπείας, ἐν αὐτῷ τῷ διακινεῖν ἐθεραπεύθη τελέως, ὡς τὸ πρᾶγμα παραπλήσιον εἶναι μαγείᾳ. (On the tendons—for I name in this way, obviously, the ends of the muscles—in addition to the aforementioned use of medicines, it is possible to see a most obvious improvement if someone uses well the therapy through the pyrite stone. It is necessary, having made it red hot, to sprinkle it with the most sour vinegar, then to move the affected limb over the stone, so that the growth may be dissolved through the vapor rising up. For many [limbs that were] once completely angled and crooked were completely cured through this kind of therapy in the very movement [of the limbs over the stone], so that the matter is very close to magic.) I thank Dr. Charles Burnett for his help in translating the Greek text.

55. See Bos, "R. Moshe Narboni," 225. Cf. *Moreh nevukhim* 3.57. For the dictum of the Sages, see TB *Shabbath* 67a; Urbach, *The Sages,* 1:101; Veltri, *Magie und Halakha,* 221 ff.

56. See Steinschneider, *Verzeichniss der hebräischen Handschriften,* MS no. 233; Steinschneider, "Eine altfranzösische Compilation," 401.

57. Cf. *Medical Aphorisms* 10.56 (ed. Bos). Salmias quotes from the Hebrew translation composed by Nathan ha-Me'ati. For Salmias of Lunel, cf. Gross, *Gallia Judaica: Dictionnaire géographique,* 288–89, no. 25.

58. Cf. Renan, *Les écrivains juifs français,* 438.

59. Cf. Steinschneider, *Verzeichniss der hebräischen Handschriften,* MS no. 113 (p. 93), fol. 35a.

60. *Shut Maharshakh* 2.105.

61. See Conrad, review of "Medical and Paramedical Manuscripts," 136–37.

62. Cf. García-Ballester, "The New Galen," 58.

63. Maimonides, *Pirke Mosheh,* ed. Muntner, x. Muntner adds that for the most difficult passages, he also consulted the Arabic text of **G**.

64. See the supplement for a concrete impression of the degree of corruption of Muntner's edition. For a similar conclusion regarding Muntner's edition of *Bi-refu'at ha-teḥorim,* see Bos, "Ibn al-Jazzār on Sexuality," 264–66.

65. Ullmann, "Zwei spätantike Kommentare," 249 n. 21.

66. See Barkaï, *Les infortunes de Dinah,* 8 n. 1: "La faiblesse principale des textes de Fred Rosner sur la médecine de Maimonide réside dans le fait qu'il ignore la médecine du temps, grecque, musulmane, et chrétienne" (The principal weakness of Fred Rosner's texts on the medical work of Maimonides lies in the fact that he is unfamiliar with the medical practice of the time—Greek, Muslim, and Christian).

67. Text between brackets in Muntner's edition of the Hebrew translation by Nathan are additions by the editor. For Nathan's translation itself, I have consulted MS Paris, BN héb. 1173 (פ), dating from the fourteenth century (see Zotenberg, ed., *Catalogues des manuscrits hébreux,* 215).

68. I have consulted MS Berlin, Or. Qu 512 (ב), dating from the fifteenth century; see Steinschneider, *Verzeichniss der hebräischen Handschriften,* no. 63.

69. For the Hebrew translations of the index, I have consulted the same manuscripts as for the comparative list of the supplement. In the case of corruptions, I also consulted MS Oxford, Michigan Add. 42. See Neubauer, *Catalogue of the Hebrew Manuscripts,* no. 2117 (p. 721) for Nathan's Hebrew translation and MS Munich 111 (מ). See Steinschneider, *Die hebräischen Handschriften der K. Hof- und Staatsbibliothek,* no. 111, for the translation by Zeraḥyah.

70. Cf. Zeraḥyah's own testimony as to the use of foreign words in the introduction to his translation of the Arabic text of Galen's *De compositione medicamentorum per genera* (MS Hamburg 309, fol. 121), reproduced in Steinschneider, *Catalog der hebräischen Handschriften in der Stadtbibliothek,* 197–99; see also Bos, *Aristotle's* De Anima, 22–43, esp. 23. For a list of these Romance terms, see the special index that appears in the index volume that accompanies this edition of *Medical Aphorisms.*

71. For instance, one of the allegedly anonymous translations of Maimonides' *On Hemorrhoids* (MS Parma; cf. Richler, ed., *Hebrew Manuscripts in the Bibliotheca Palatina,* 1531, 4 fols. 20r–25v), was actually prepared by Zeraḥyah, as I will show in my forthcoming edition of this text.

72. See Pertsch, *Die orientalischen Handschriften,* 3:477–78; Kahle, "Aphorismum Praefatio et Excerpta," 89–90.

73. Other missing sections are 20.30–33 and 25.56–58.

74. See the remark by the scribe at the end of **G**, treatise 24 (fol. 239a): "Something like the following was written at the end of this treatise: This is what I found in the copy written by Abū [. . .]: I did not make a fair copy of this treatise until after his death, may God have mercy with him; and [A]bū al-Zakāt the physician wrote: Praise be to God, who is exalted."

75. See Pertsch, *Die orientalischen Handschriften,* 3:477–78; Kahle, "Aphorismum Praefatio et Excerpta," 90; Kaufmann, "Le neveu de Maïmonide," 152–53; Sirat, "Une liste de manuscrits," 112; Meyerhof, "Medical Work," 276; Kraemer, "Six Unpublished Maimonides Letters," 79–80 n. 93; Stern, "Maimonides' Treatise to a Prince," 18.

76. See Schacht and Meyerhof, "Maimonides against Galen," 59; *Aphorisms,* trans. Rosner, xiv.

77. See Voorhoeve, comp., *Handlist of Arabic Manuscripts,* 85.

78. See Dozy, *Supplément aux dictionnaires arabes,* 1:836; Kahle, "Aphorismum Praefatio et Excerpta," 90–91.

79. Zotenberg, *Catalogues des manuscrits hébreux,* 223; Vajda, *Index général des manuscrits arabes musulmans,* 345.

80. See Derenbourg and Renaud, *Médecine et histoire naturelle,* 74–75; Ledesma, *Manuscritos árabes de El Escorial,* 65, no. 33.

81. See Derenbourg and Renaud, *Médecine et histoire naturelle,* 76; Ledesma, *Manuscritos árabes de El Escorial,* 65, no. 33.

82. See Neubauer, *Catalogue of the Hebrew Manuscripts,* no. 2113 (p. 721); see also Beit-Arié and May, *Supplement,* col. 392.

83. Beit-Arié and May, *Supplement,* col. 392, states that Steinschneider refers to "a physician by the name of Makhluf of Marsala, Syracuse (Sicily)."

84. Galen, *De usu partium* 12.3 (ed. Helmreich, 2:188 line 4).

85. See Neubauer, *Catalogue of the Hebrew Manuscripts,* no. 2114 (p. 721); Beit-Arié and May, *Supplement,* col. 392.

86. See Neubauer, *Catalogue of the Hebrew Manuscripts,* no. 2115 (p. 721); Beit-Arié and May, *Supplement,* col. 392.

87. See Kahle, "Aphorismum Praefatio et Excerpta," 89.

88. See Ullmann, *Medizin im Islam,* 167, no. 4. I was unable to obtain photocopies of this manuscript.

89. Meyerhof, "Medical Work," 272.

90. Blau, *Background of Judaeo-Arabic,* 41; see Baron, *Philosophy and Science,* 403 n. 42.

91. "Maimonides' Treatise to a Prince," ed. and trans. Stern, 18; see also Blau, *Background of Judaeo-Arabic,* 41.

92. Langermann, "Arabic Writings in Hebrew Manuscripts," 139.

93. Ibn Sahl, *Dispensatorium parvum,* ed. Kahl, 35–38.

Author's Introduction

Unless otherwise indicated, all translations of quotations in the notes are my own.

1. Kahle, "Aphorismum Praefatio et Excerpta," 91, translates this as "Geisteswissenschaften," or "humanities." In comparison, see Efros, *Philosophical Terms,* 66, s.v. "limmudim": "mathematical science, particularly astronomy; Ar. *al-taᶜālīm.*"

2. By "perfect languages," Maimonides probably means those languages spoken by the inhabitants of the temperate climatic zones. Following the theory propounded by al-Fārābī in his *Kitāb al-ḥurūf* that the faculties of man are influenced by the physical conditions of the environment, Maimonides remarks in *Medical Aphorisms* 25.58 (ed. Bos) that, since these inhabitants "have more perfect intellects and better forms; that is, their shape and outline is more regular, their organs are better proportioned, and their temperament is more balanced than that of the inhabitants of the distant climatic zones in the extreme north and south, so the pronunciation of the letters by the inhabitants of the temperate climatic zones and the movement of their speech organs during speaking is more balanced and closer to human articulated speech than the pronunciation of the letters and the movement of the speech organs of those [people], I mean, the inhabitants of the distant climatic zones in the extreme [north and south] and their language." Examples of these "perfect" languages are, according to Maimonides, Greek, Hebrew, Arabic, Persian, and Aramaic; see my edition of *Medical Aphorisms* 22–25. See also Zwiep, *Mother of Reason,* 194–97.

3. See Maimonides, *On Asthma* 13.49 (ed. Bos, 109): "Rather, this art is difficult for most scholars not with respect to understanding it, but with respect to remembering it, because it requires [the command of] a very large amount of memorized material."

4. See Hippocrates, *Aphorisms* (ed. Littré, 4:396–609; trans. Jones, 4:98–221).

5. Al-Rāzī, *Kitāb al-murshid aw al-fuṣūl.* Al-Rāzī (865–932) was one of the foremost Arab physicians and "the most freethinking of the major philosophers." See EI^2, 8:474–77, s.v. "al-Rāzī" (Goodman). Maimonides quotes from these aphorisms in his treatise On Asthma 13.8, 12 (ed. Bos, 84, 87). See as well *Medical Aphorisms* 25.1 (ed. Bos) for Maimonides' defense of Galen against the criticism of al-Rāzī.

6. ʿAbd Allāh ibn Muḥammad al-Taqafī al-Sūsī (942–1012), known as Abū Muḥammad, a physician who took up residence in Córdoba, where he was killed by Berbers. Al-Sūsī is quoted twice in the *Kitāb al-wisād* of Ibn Wāfid from Toledo (see Alvarez de Morales y Ruiz-Matas, trans., "El Libro de la Almohada," 3.128 [p. 102] and 15.13 [p. 236]. For bibliographical details, see p. 102 n. 12).

7. Yūḥannā ibn Māsawayh, *Le livre des axiomes médicaux,* ed. and trans. Jacquart and Troupeau. Ibn Māsawayh (777–857) was hospital director and physician to the caliphs.

8. Abū Naṣr al-Fārābī (870?–950), "one of the most outstanding and renowned Muslim philosophers"; see EI^2, 2:778–81, s.v. "al-Fārābī" (Walzer).

9. "And I do not claim . . . the idea that Galen mentioned": For this section I have closely followed the translation in Langermann, "Synochous Fever," 177.

10. **ELBP** read "certain."

11. **EL** have "the meanings of [certain] nomina," reading مدلولات *(madlūlāt)* as مداولات *(mudāwalāt);* Kahle, "Aphorismum Praefatio et Excerpta," 93, translates it as "Diskussionen."

12. Literally, "waters."

The First Treatise

1. Galen, *De usu partium* 7.14 (ed. Helmreich, 1:413; trans. May, 1:361). The missing part, vital for the understanding of the next sentence, reads thus: "Nerves like those of the diaphragm that are inserted into the middle of a muscle and distributed from that point to all parts of it draw all the fibers toward the center."

2. See Galen, *De usu partium* 13.5 (ed. Helmreich, 2:256 lines 4–5): ἡ κεφαλὴ δέ, ἐφ' ἣν ἀναρτῶνται τοῖς μυσὶν ἅπασιν αἱ ἶνες. Trans. May, 2:600, reads this as "Its head, the point to which in all muscles the fibers are attached. . . ."

3. In trans. May, 2:600, this missing section reads "For with the diaphragm as it actually is, it was necessary to have the head of the muscle either at its center or at the parts that are opposite the center."

4. See the Greek text in Galen, *De usu partium* 13.5 (ed. Helmreich, 2:256): τὸν περιγράφοντα κύκλον ὅλον αὐτοῦ; see also trans. May, 2:600, which reads "and describes a complete circle."

5. Galen, *De usu partium* 13.5 (ed. Helmreich, 2:256; trans. May, 2:600). For the Arabic translation by Ḥubaysh, revised by Ḥunayn, see MS Paris 2853, fols. 235b–236a.

6. Literally, "are attached to."

7. Added according to MS Paris 2853, fol. 157a; see also the Greek text in Galen, *De usu partium* 9.5 (ed. Helmreich, 2:15): τὰ δεόμενα τῶν ἀγγείων ἀμφοτέρων. Trans. May, 1:434, reads this as "needing both kinds of vessels."

8. "With the sole exception of the brain": This portion is missing in the Greek text; see Galen, *De usu partium* 9.5 (ed. Helmreich, 2:15–18).

9. Literally, "streaming."

10. See Galen, *De usu partium* 9.5 (ed. Helmreich, 2:15–18; trans. May, 1:434–36).

11. The archaic terms *coct* and *coction,* from the same root as the word *cook,* were used in humoralist theory to designate either the digestion of food, the processing of bodily humors into a more easily assimilated state, or a normal heating or processing stage in the healing of a wound or the course of a disease.

12. Galen, *De usu partium* 16.10 (ed. Helmreich, 2:419; trans. May, 2:712); MS Paris 2853, fol. 290b; trans. Savage-Smith, 92, 170–71.

13. MS Paris 2853, fol. 290b, reads thus: فليس بالعجب أن يكون ما يأتي العظام من العروق غير الضوارب صغار تخفى عن البصر (So one should not be surprised that veins so small that they are hidden from the eye reach the bones.) Compare Galen, *De usu partium* 16.14 (ed. Helmreich, 2:433; trans. May, 2:722).

14. Galen, *De usu partium* 16.14 (ed. Helmreich, 2:433–35; trans. May, 2:722).

15. **SGB** literally read "if the species of nerves is stretched"; **EL** read "if the body of the nerve is stretched." Galen, *De causis pulsum* 2.12 (ed. Kühn, 9:89), actually reads ἐν τῷ διαστέλλεσθαι τὰς ἀρτηρίας (when the arteries are stretched).

16. Galen's *De pulsu [magna] (Megapulsus)* encompasses four books, consisting of four treatises each, for a total of sixteen treatises: *De differentia pulsuum,*

De dignoscendis pulsibus, De causis pulsuum, and *De praesagitione ex pulsibus.* Maimonides' quote appears in *De caus. puls.,* 2.12 (ed. Kühn, 9:88–90), which is the tenth treatise of *De pulsu [magna].* See Ullmann, *Medizin im Islam,* 43, no. 31; Steinschneider, "Griechischen Ärzte," 282 (334).

17. Galen, *De methodo medendi* 6.4 (ed. Kühn, 10:409).

18. Galen, *De usu partium* 16.2 (ed. Helmreich, 2:379–82; trans. May, 2:683–85); trans. Savage-Smith, 59–61, 111–15.

19. See Galen, *De motu musculorum* 1.2 (ed. Kühn, 4:374). Trans. Goss, 3, reads this as "the bulk of."

20. Trans. Goss, 3, translates this as "binding tissue"; see also 24–25, where he points to the varying meanings of the Greek equivalent σύνδεσμος.

21. Literally, "because of the amount of ligament mixed with it."

22. See Galen, *De motu musculorum* 1.2 (ed. Kühn, 4:374; trans. Goss, 3). The Arabic title *Fī ḥarakāt al-ᶜaḍal* actually means *De motibus musculorum.*

23. Literally, "organs" or "instruments." Trans. Savage-Smith, 43, renders it as "systems" in the case of nerves, veins, and arteries.

24. *Mutaqāriba al-ḥāl:* "similar," corresponding to the Greek παραπλήσια in ed. de Lacy, 94 line 11.

25. Literally, "they mostly become so wide"; cf. ed. de Lacy, 94: πλατύνονται γὰρ οἱ πλείους αὐτῶν. Cf. **B**.

26. Galen, *De placitis Hippocratis et Platonis* 1.9.1–3 (ed. de Lacy, 94–95).

27. Ibid.

28. In Greek, εὐθείας. Galen, *De placitis Hippocratis et Platonis* 1.9.8 (ed. de Lacy, 96 line1).

29. Galen, *De placitis Hippocratis et Platonis* 1.9.8 (ed. de Lacy, 96 line1).

30. Galen, *De motu musculorum* 1.1 (ed. Kühn, 4:373; trans. Goss, 3). Maimonides' reference (*fī tilka al-maqāla* [ibidem]) is incorrect, since he is not referring to the previous source citation but to the source cited before it. It is, however, possible that the order of the paragraphs was originally different.

31. Trans. Goss, 3, uses "fascia"; see n. 19 above.

32. In Greek, διαφύσεις. Galen, *De motu musculorum* 1.1 (ed. Kühn, 4.371). The term is not rendered in trans. Goss.

33. Galen, *De motu musculorum* 1.1 (ed. Kühn, 4:371; trans. Goss, 3).

34. Galen, *De motu musculorum* 1.3 (ed. Kühn, 4:377–78; trans. Goss, 4).

35. In Greek, ἐμφράξεις. Galen, *De alimentorum facultatibus* 3.15 (ed. Kühn, 6:687; ed. Helmreich, 348 line 12).

36. Galen, *De alimentorum facultatibus* 3.15 (ed. Kühn, 6:687; ed. Helmreich, 348 lines 12–15).

37. Galen, *De alimentorum facultatibus* 3.16 (ed. Kühn, 6:693; ed. Helmreich, 351 line 28–352 line 4).

38. Galen, *De usu partium* 2.7 (ed. Helmreich, 1:86–87; trans. May, 1:130).

39. *Juzʾān:* "two parts"; MS Paris 2853 reads "can be found" *(mawjūdān).*

40. See Galen, *De usu partium* 6.10 (ed. Helmreich, 1:328; trans. May, 1:299).

41. See Galen, *De usu partium* 6.10 (ed. Helmreich, 1:332; trans. May, 1:303).

42. Galen, *De usu pulsuum* 5 (ed. Kühn, 5:166; English translation found in *On Respiration and the Arteries,* ed. and trans. Furley and Wilkie, 212–13). Galen's

De usu pulsuum was also known under the Arabic title *Maqāla fī al-ḥāja ilā al-nabḍ;* see Ullmann, *Medizin im Islam,* 41, no. 16.

43. *Muḥkam:* "completely." The Greek equivalent is ἀκριβῶς, meaning, literally, "exactly." See Galen, *De naturalibus facultatibus* 3.14 (ed. Kühn, 2:205; trans. Brock, 316–17).

44. Galen, *De naturalibus facultatibus* 3.14 (ed. Kühn, 2:205; trans. Brock, 316–17).

45. Perhaps the breasts, i.e., the twofold thoracic cavity.

46. The title of this lost treatise attributed to Galen can be found in a list compiled by the Arab bibliographer Ibn Abī Uṣaybiʿa (Steinschneider, "Griechischen Ärzte," 461 [355], no. 102; Max Meyerhof, "Schriften Galens," 543). It is not identical with "Galen's Commentary on Hippocrates' *Diaites Hygienes,*" as suggested by *Aphorisms,* trans. Rosner, 9, following Maimonides, *Pirḳe Mosheh,* ed. Muntner, 402, no. 15.

47. Galen, *De usu partium* 11.10 (ed. Helmreich, 2:141; trans. May, 2:522).

48. See MS Paris 2853, fol. 278b, which reads "and in its other characteristics—apart from its thickness—it is similar to it."

49. MS Paris 2853, fol. 278b, adds "at first sight."

50. MS Paris 2853, fol. 278b, reads thus: "But when you dissect it, you know for certain that it is not."

51. Galen, *De usu partium* 16.5 (ed. Helmreich, 2:395–96; trans. May, 2:695).

52. *Yanfatil:* after the Greek μεταφέρονται. Galen, *De motu musculorum* 1.8 (ed. Kühn, 4:403). Trans. Goss, 10, has "carried about."

53. Galen, *De motu musculorum* 1.8 (ed. Kühn, 4:403–4; trans. Goss, 10).

54. Goss uses the term "antagonistic" muscles in his translation of Galen's *De motu musculorum.* See *The New Oxford Dictionary of the English Language,* s.v. "antagonistic": "Anatomy: A muscle whose action counteracts that of another specified muscle."

55. Literally, "remains."

56. Literally, "contracted."

57. Galen, *De motu musculorum* 1.4, 5 (ed. Kühn, 4:387–88; trans. Goss, 6–7).

58. Galen, *De motu musculorum* 2.4 (ed. Kühn, 4:435; trans. Goss, 17).

59. Galen, *De motu musculorum* 2.8 (ed. Kühn, 4:454–58; trans. Goss, 22–23).

60. Galen, *De motu musculorum* 2.9 (ed. Kühn, 4:461; trans. Goss, 24).

61. Translated according to **LBP**.

62. Galen, *De motu musculorum* 2.9 (ed. Kühn, 4:459; trans. Goss, 23).

63. In Galen, *De motu musculorum* 1.10 (ed. Kühn, 4:420), the Greek reads: ἄλλοτ' ἄλλου σχήματος ὀρέγεται. Trans. Goss, 14, has "pull themselves about from one position to another."

64. Galen, *De motu musculorum* 1.10 (ed. Kühn, 4:420; trans. Goss, 14).

65. Galen, *De locis affectis* 5.1 (ed. Kühn, 8:300; trans. Siegel, 137).

66. Galen, *De motu musculorum* 2.5 (ed. Kühn, 4:440–41; trans. Goss, 19).

67. The Arabic expression *ḥalla al-shakk* is reminiscent of the title *Ḥallu shukūk al-Rāzī* (To resolve the doubts raised by al-Rāzī). It refers to a number of works composed by several Islamic physicians—as, for instance, ʿAlī ibn Riḍwān (d. 1068), Abū al-ʿAlāʾ ibn āuhr (d. 1130–31), and ʿAbd al-Laṭīf al-Baghdādī

(d. 1231–32) who, just like Maimonides in *Medical Aphorisms* 25.1 (ed. Bos), came to the defense of Galen against the attack by al-Rāzī (865–932) in his *Kitāb al-shukūk ʿalā Jālīnūs.* See Averroës, "Averroes 'contra Galenum," ed. and trans. Bürgel, 285; this source notes that the term *shukūk* is a parallel to the Greek πρόβλημα, ζήτημα, or ἀπορία.

68. On the role of imagination in causing an erection, see Ibn al-Jazzār, *Sexual Diseases,* ed. and trans. Bos, 22, 240.

69. This is the technical term, rendered thus by Pines in his translation of the *Moreh nevukhim* (Pines, trans., *The Guide of the Perplexed,* 2:610).

70. Galen, *De motu musculorum* 2.4 (ed. Kühn, 4:439), reads οὐ γὰρ ἀναίσθητοι παντάπασίν εἰσιν οἱ ὑπνώττοντες, ἀλλὰ δυσαίσθητοι. Trans. Goss, 18, has "For those sleeping are not entirely without sensation, although they sense with difficulty."

71. Aristotle describes the different processes involved in the activity of motion in detail in his *Movement of Animals.* Motion requires that the "affections fittingly prepare the organic parts, the desire prepares the affections, and the imagination prepares the desire, while the imagination [itself] is due to thought or sensation." Aristotle, *Movement of Animals* 8.702a18 ff. (trans. Forster, 466–67).

72. Galen, *De motu musculorum* 2.6 (ed. Kühn, 4:445–46; trans. Goss, 20).

73. See Aristotle, *De memoria* 453a5 ff. (trans. Hett, 308–11); see also the summary in Averroës, *Epitome of* Parva naturalia, ed. and trans. Blumberg, 86 n. 4.

74. Galen, *De motu musculorum* 2.4 (ed. Kühn, 4:436–39; trans. Goss, 18).

75. Compare Galen, *De instrumento odoratus* 32.4 (ed. and trans. Kollesch as *Galen über das Riechorgan,* 33.4). The translation reads "Tatsächlich zeigt es sich bei den Säuglingen, oder wenn ein Schädel aufgebohrt ist, dass sich das Gehirn beim Einatmen hebt und ausdehnt, dass es aber beim Ausatmen zusammenschrumpft und sich kontrahiert" (Indeed, we see in the case of infants or of trepanation of the skull that, with inhalation, the brain raises and expands itelf, but with exhalation shrinks and contracts).

76. This second part of Maimonides' quotation has no parallel in the source given, which has not been preserved in the Arabic tradition (see *Ḥunain ibn Isḥāq,* ed. and trans. Bergsträsser, no. 48; Sezgin, *Medizin-Pharmazie-Zoologie-Tierheilkunde* 3:106 no. 39). *Galen über das Riechorgan,* ed. and trans. Kollesch, 23, does not address the quotations from this text appearing in Maimonides' *Medical Aphorisms.*

77. That is, the *pia mater.*

78. That is, the *dura mater.*

79. The Arabic text reads according to the Greek version in Galen, *De usu partium* 8.9 (ed. Helmreich, 478 lines 7–8): καὶ γὰρ δὴ καὶ ἀφέστηκεν ἀπ' αὐτῆς ἡ παχεῖα (the thick [membrane] is separated from it), where αὐτῆς, the feminine form of "it," refers to the thin membrane; however, a better reading is provided in Kühn's edition, 3:659: καὶ γὰρ δὴ καὶ ἀφέστηκεν ἀπ' αὐτοῦ ἡ παχεῖα (the thick [membrane] is separated from it), where αὐτοῦ, the masculine form of "it," refers to the brain. See trans. May, 1:410, and n. 57.

80. Maimonides is referring to the *lamina cribrosa.*

81. Galen, *De usu partium* 8.6–9 (ed. Helmreich, 1:472–78; trans. May, 1:407–11).

82. That is, the *retiform plexus,* or "rete mirabile," the network of blood vessels Galen apparently observed at the base of the bovine brain and assumed was also present in humans.

83. Galen, *De usu partium* 9.4 (ed. Helmreich, 2:10–15; trans. May, 1:430–34).

84. Galen, *De usu partium* 8.8 (ed. Helmreich, 2:262–64; trans. May, 2:604–5).

85. "Requires a more exact discrimination": cf. Galen, *De locis affectis* 4.3 (ed. Kühn, 8:229; trans. Siegel, 109): ὡς ἂν ἀκριβεστέρας δεομένη διαγνώσεως.

86. Galen, *De locis affectis* 4.3 (ed. Kühn, 8:229; trans. Siegel, 109).

87. Galen, *De locis affectis* 4.6 (ed. Kühn, 8:241; trans. Siegel, 114).

88. Galen, *De locis affectis* 4.9 (ed. Kühn, 8:266–67; trans. Siegel, 124).

89. Galen, *De usu partium* 10.6 (ed. Helmreich, 2:74–78; trans. May, 2:478–79).

90. **E** adds "in its movements."

91. The Greek original of this text by Galen and the Arabic translation by Ḥubaysh are lost; the text survives only in a Latin translation; see Sezgin, *Medizin-Pharmazie-Zoologie-Tierheilkunde,* 100, no. 23; Ullmann, *Medizin im Islam,* 54, no. 75.

92. The Arabic term for *tremore,* as quoted by Sezgin, *Medizin-Pharmazie-Zoologie-Tierheilkunde,* 135, no. 139, is *riʿsha* instead of *riʿda.*

93. Galen, *De tremore, palpitatione, convulsione, et rigore* 2 (ed. Kühn, 7:585). This is the only quotation known from the Arabic translation by Ḥubaysh; see Sezgin, *Medizin-Pharmazie-Zoologie-Tierheilkunde,* 135, no. 139.

94. That is, Galen.

95. Cf. Galen, *De naturalibus facultatibus* 3.13 (ed. Kühn, 2:188–89, 197; trans. Brock, 292–93, 304–5).

96. *ʿUnuq:* literally, "neck." In the case of the bladder, it is indeed the neck which carries out the attraction and elimination of the food.

97. Cf. Galen, *De naturalibus facultatibus* 3.13 (ed. Kühn, 2:188 lines 4–5; trans Brock, 290): τούτου δ' ἔτι μᾶλλον οὐ χρὴ θαυμάζειν.

98. Literally, "the stomach and what is connected to it."

99. That is, the mesenteric veins.

100. Literally, "stomach."

101. Galen, *De naturalibus facultatibus* 3.13 (ed. Kühn 2:187–89; trans. Brock, 290–93).

102. Galen, *De usu partium* 3.5 (ed. Helmreich, 1:137). Trans. May, 1:162–63, has "Locomotion is accomplished by support and motion, and the foot is the instrument of one element and the whole leg of the other." Cf. MS Paris 2853, fol. 44a.

103. Galen, *De usu partium* 6.9 (ed. Helmreich, 1:322; trans. May, 1:295).

104. "It is flat" مسطوحة: The Greek equivalent is ἐντετύπωται, which is rendered in trans. May, 1:210 as "it molds itself upon them" (meaning the vertebrae).

105. That is, the omentum.

106. Galen, *De usu partium* 4.7–8 (ed. Helmreich, 1:204–8; trans. May, 1:210–14).

107. Galen, *De usu partium* 4.9 (ed. Helmreich, 1:209; trans. May, 1:214).

108. That is, the peritoneum.

109. Galen, *De usu partium* 4.10 (ed. Helmreich, 1:215; trans. May, 1:218–19).

110. Galen, *De usu partium* 4.19 (ed. Helmreich, 1:247; trans. May, 1:242).

111. Galen, *De naturalibus facultatibus* 3.7 (ed. Kühn 2:161; trans. Brock, 250–51).

112. "Passed to": according to the Greek προστιθεμένην. Galen, *De naturalibus facultatibus* 3.13 (ed. Kühn 2:200). I have adopted the translation in trans. Brock, 309. The Arabic equivalent يزيد literally means "added to."

113. Galen, *De naturalibus facultatibus* 3.13 (ed. Kühn 12:200–202; trans. Brock, 308–11).

114. Galen's *De morborum causis et symptomatibus* consists of six books: *De morborum differentiis, De causis morborum liber, De symptomatum differentiis liber,* and *De symptomatum causis* 1–3 (see Ullmann, *Medizin im Islam,* 42, no. 22). The designation of book 6 given here refers, therefore, to *De symptomatum causis* 3. See Galen, *De symptomatum causis* 3.4 (ed. Kühn, 7:224–25): "The first and actually most necessary of all the natural activities is nutrition, which is a kind of alteration. For the concoction in the stomach is an alteration, and likewise that in the veins and that in all the [other parts], in which there is a fourth alteration, called 'assimilation.' And although this name is different from that of nutrition, it refers to the same activity."

115. Literally, "fat," meaning the layer of fat surrounding the stomach. See 1.54 of translated text and n. 105 of this treatise.

116. Galen, *De methodo medendi* 6.4 (ed. Kühn, 10:423).

117. Literally, "body."

118. Galen, *De usu partium* 4.15 (ed. Helmreich, 1:232–33; trans. May, 1:232–33).

119. Cf. Galen, *De usu partium* 5.5 (ed. Helmreich, 1:266). Trans. May, 1:256, reads "It is also proper to understand the usefulness of the way in which the kidneys are placed, that is, the reason . . . why the right one is higher up and frequently attached to the liver itself, and the left one is lower than the right." As May remarks in n. 20: "Galen's sensible arguments . . . are all nullified by the fact that in man the left kidney is usually the higher of the two. He was almost certainly describing conditions in some species of ape." By adding "in some living beings," Maimonides has thus correctly limited the validity of Galen's general statement.

120. Galen, *De usu partium* 5.6 (ed. Helmreich, 1:269; trans. May, 1:258).

121. The correct reference is *De usu partium* 5, ed. Helmreich, 1:266; see also trans. May, 1:256. In book 4, Galen only remarks that "the right kidney [lies] higher up for a reason which I shall give later on." See Galen, *De usu partium* 4.18 (ed. Helmreich, 1:245); see also trans. May, 1:241.

122. Galen, *De usu partium* 5.7–8 (ed. Helmreich, 1:273–75; trans. May, 1:261–62).

123. Galen, *De usu partium* 14.3 (ed. Helmreich, 2:287; trans. May, 2:623).

124. "Two uteri": cf. trans. May, 2:260 n. 2: "Galen was following well-established custom when he usually (though not always) employed the plural in speaking of the uterus. He was thinking, of course, of the bi-cornate uterus as two organs having a common outlet. . . ."

125. Galen, *De usu partium* 14.4 (ed. Helmreich, 2:292; trans. May, 2:626).

126. Galen, *De usu partium* 14.4 (ed. Helmreich, 2:291; trans. May, 2:625).

127. Literally, "closer to the type of sinews," or "more nervelike." The Greek term is νευρωδεστέρα.

128. Galen, *De praes. ex puls.* 4.7 (ed. Kühn, 9:404).

129. Galen, *De naturalibus facultatibus* 1.6 and 3.11 (ed. Kühn 2:13–15, 180–82; trans. Brock, 22–25, 281–83); see also Galen, *De usu partium* 6.11, 12 (ed. Helmreich, 1:333, 341; trans. May, 1:304, 310).

130. Galen, *De usu partium* 15.2–3 (ed. Helmreich, 2:343–45; trans. May, 2:659–60).

131. That is, the peritoneum; see section 1.56 above.

132. Galen, *De usu partium* 5.9–11 (ed. Helmreich, 1:276, 281; trans. May, 1:263, 266).

133. Literally, "bodies."

134. Galen, *De praesagitione ex pulsibus* 4.7 (ed. Kühn, 9:404–5).

135. Arabic *yad* can also mean "arm."

136. **EL** read "organs."

137. Literally, they swell or protrude.

138. Rosner, trans., *Aphorisms,* translates this as "semimaximally."

139. Literally, "bodies."

140. Galen, *De motu musculorum* 1.3 (ed. Kühn, 4:380–82; trans. Goss, 5).

141. Galen, *De motu musculorum* 1.3 (ed. Kühn, 4:379–80; trans. Goss, 4–5).

142. That is, the elementary tissues; also called "homoiomerous" (ὁμοιομερής). These are as Peter Brain remarks in *Galen on bloodletting,* 8: ". . . substances such as bone, flesh, and the humours which have no naked-eye structure. They are formed from the four elements, which however are so mixed in them that none is individually perceptible." This concept already features in Aristotle, *De partibus animalium* 2.1.646a8–647a8. Cf. trans. May, 1:67 n. 2.

143. Galen, *De naturalibus facultatibus* 1.6 (ed. Kühn 2:15; trans. Brock, 24–25) calls this faculty τεχνική (artistic). It is possible that the Arabic عقلي is a corruption of عملي.

144. Galen, *De naturalibus facultatibus* 1.5, 6–11 (ed. Kühn 2:10–26; trans. Brock, 18–43).

145. Galen, *De naturalibus facultatibus* 1.7 (ed. Kühn 2:16; trans. Brock, 26–27).

146. Galen, *De naturalibus facultatibus* 3.11 (ed. Kühn 2:180–81; trans. Brock, 280–83).

The Second Treatise

1. Galen distinguishes blood qua humor and blood qua the substance found in the veins and arteries. One is pure, almost a concept; the other, a mixture of humors (personal communication from Vivian Nutton).

2. Galen, *In Hippocratis Epidemiarum Libros I et II* (ed. Wenkebach and Pfaff, 342 lines 15–27). See also trans. Deller, 525 n. 26. The fourteenth-century French surgeon Guy de Chauliac refers to the Latin translation of this text in his *Inventarium sive chirurgia magna* 1:60 lines 39–40; 2:59.

3. غسالة: Cf. Lane, *Arabic-English Lexicon,* 2:2259: "That with which one has washed the thing. . . . The infusion of the thing. . . . What is extracted from the thing by washing." Also compare the Greek περίχυμα, in Galen, *In Hippocratis Epidemiarum* 6.1–8 (ed. Wenkebach and Pfaff, 109 line 5).

4. That is, blood serum. The Greek term is ὀρρός τε και ἰχώρ. Galen, *In Hippocratis Epidemiarum* 6.1–8 (ed. Wenkebach and Pfaff, 109 line 12).

5. Galen, *In Hippocratis Epidemiarum* 6.1–8 (Wenkebach and Pfaff, 109 lines 4–11); see also trans. Deller, 535 n. 73.

6. Cf. the Greek in Galen, *De atra bile* 2 (ed. Kühn, 5:109; ed. de Boer, 74 line 3): κἂν ὠχρά, κἂν ξανθή, κἂν λεκιθώδης φαίνηται (whether pallid, yellow, or yolk-colored).

7. Galen, *De atra bile* 2 (ed. Kühn, 5:109–10; ed. de Boer, 73–74).

8. Galen, *In Hippocratis Prognostica commentarius* 2.38–39 (ed. Kühn, 18B:165–68).

9. Galen, *In Hippocratis Epidemiarum* 6.1–8 (ed. Wenkebach and Pfaff, 25 lines 7–9). See also trans. Deller, 531 n. 57.

10. *Fī al-ḥummayāt (De febribus)* is the Arabic title for Galen's *De differentiis febrium.* Maimonides' quotation features in 2.6 (ed. Kühn, 7:348–49).

11. *Durdī:* Translation of this term as "lees of wine" reflects the Greek τρύξ, in Galen, *De naturalibus facultatibus* 2.9 (ed. Kühn 2:135). See also trans. Brock, 208–9.

12. That is, when it is healthy.

13. That is, when it becomes ill.

14. Galen, *De naturalibus facultatibus* 2.9 (ed. Kühn 2:135–38; trans. Brock, 208–13).

15. Section 8 is missing in all the Arabic manuscripts but appears in the Hebrew translations.

16. Translated according to מבפ, which have "place."

17. Galen, *De usu partium* 8.6 (ed. Helmreich, 470–71; trans. May, 406–7).

18. "I will also describe the device provided by nature": translated according to פ.

19. Namely, in Galen, *De usu partium* 5.3 (ed. Helmreich 259; trans. May, 251–52).

20. Galen, *De naturalibus facultatibus* 2.9 (trans. Brock, 214–17). This aphorism is missing in all the Arabic manuscripts and in the Latin translations (editions Bologna 1489 and Basel 1579), but appears in מבפ. My edition and translation of the Hebrew text is based on ב. In two places I have consulted פ, when ב appeared corrupt.

21. Meaning that the blood needs yellow bile.

22. Galen, *De naturalibus facultatibus* 2.9 (ed. Kühn 2:137–39; trans. Brock, 212–15).

23. Cf. Galen, *De naturalibus facultatibus* 2.9 (ed. Kühn 2:140). Trans. Brock, 216–17, reads "in accordance with its nature."

24. Literally, "coction." According to *Maimonides' Regimen of Health,* ed. and trans. Bar-Sela, Hoff, and Faris, 17 n. 10, "Galen explained the physiology of

nutrition in terms of three orders of digestion [or coction], the first . . . taking place in the stomach, the second in the liver—the major nutritive organ where the food is turned into blood—and the third in the rest of the organs which the nutriments reach via the veins." See also Galen, *In Hippocratis De alimento commentarius* 2.3 (ed. Kühn, 15:234–35); Galen, *De bon. mal. sucis* 5.17–18 (ed. Helmreich, 411); *Maimonides on the Causes of Symptoms,* ed. Leibowitz and Marcus, 61 (135v); and Maimonides, *On Asthma* 2.1 (ed. Bos, 8–9).

25. Galen, *De naturalibus facultatibus* 2.9 (ed. Kühn 2:140; trans. Brock, 216–17).

26. Galen, *De alimentorum facultatibus* 1.1 (ed. Helmreich, 207 lines 9–14).

27. Literally, "strength."

28. "Each of these humors often streams into organs while it is pure, unadulterated, and unmixed"; cf. *Medical Aphorisms* 25.38 (ed. Bos).

29. Galen, *De causis morborum* 6 (ed. Kühn, 7:21–22).

30. Galen, *De morborum differentiis* 2 (ed. Kühn, 6:839). Cf. n. 114 of treatise 1.

31. "Of diverse [categories and] types": the Greek text reads διαφοραὶ μεγάλαι . . . εἰσι κατὰ. Galen, *De locis affectis* 3.9 (ed. Kühn, 8:175–76). Trans. Siegel, 87, reads "great differences exist between."

32. Galen, *De locis affectis* 3.9 (ed. Kühn, 8:175–76; trans. Siegel, 87).

33. "Cause the ground to effervesce": the Greek reads ζυμοῖ τὴν γῆν. Galen, *De atra bile* 3 (ed. Kühn, 5:111; ed. de Boer, 74 line 22).

34. Galen, *De atra bile* 3 (ed. Kühn, 5:110–11; ed. de Boer, 74–75).

35. Galen, *De locis affectis* 3.9 (ed. Kühn, 8:176–77; trans. Siegel, 87–88).

36. Galen, *De alimentorum facultatibus* 3.1 (ed. Helmreich, 333 line 5) reads ψώρα.

37. That is, leprosy. See Galen, *De alimentorum facultatibus* 3.1 (ed. Helmreich, 333 line 5): λέπρα.

38. *Waswās:* See Lane, *Arabic-English Lexicon,* 2:2940: "A certain disease (i.e., melancholia, in which is a doting in the imagination and judgment, a sort of delirium . . .) arising from a predominance of the black bile, attended with confusion of the intellect." Cf. Galen, *De alimentorum facultatibus* 3.1 (ed. Helmreich, 333 line 5): ἥ τ' ἰδίως ὀνομαζομένη μελαγχολία. Dols, *Majnūn: The Madman,* 50, translates the term *al-waswās al-sawdāwī* as "melancholic delusion."

39. Galen, *De alimentorum facultatibus* 3.1 (ed. Helmreich, 333 line 5).

40. Galen, *De alimentorum facultatibus* 1.2 (ed. Helmreich, 221 lines 13–14) reads ἐξ ὠμῶν πλήθους.

41. Galen, *De alimentorum facultatibus* 1.2 (ed. Helmreich, 221 lines 9–16).

42. Galen, *De crisibus* 1.12 (ed. Kühn, 9:601–2).

43. Galen, *De causis pulsum* 4.26 (ed. Kühn, 9:202–3). Cf. n. 16 of treatise 1. The arterial movement is both smaller in duration and, when you put your finger on the pulse, it feels as if there is very little "give"; i.e., it is more solid throughout the movement. Even today this usually understood to indicate some kind of heart and vascular problem (personal communication from Vivian Nutton).

44. "In the cavity of the lining of the stomach": cf. the Greek text in Galen, *De compositione medicamentorum secundum locos* 2.1 (ed. Kühn, 12:539): ἐν τῷ κύτει . . . ὅλης τῆς γαστρὸς (in the cavity of the whole stomach).

45. Galen, *De compositione medicamentorum secundum locos* 2.1 (ed. Kühn, 12:538–39). For the Arabic *miyāmir,* coined after the Syriac *mēmrā* (discourse), see Ullmann, *Medizin im Islam,* 48, no. 50.

46. *Fa-yaḥbisuhu al-insān wa-yastakrihuhu:* a translation of the Greek βιαίως ἐπισχεθεὶς, in Galen, *De symptomatum causis* 3.2 (ed. Kühn, 7:219).

47. Galen, *De symptomatum causis* 3.2 (ed. Kühn, 7:219–20).

48. Galen speaks of "chyme," i.e., the fluidic substance resulting from digested food (Greek χυμὸς), not of "food"; see Galen, *De causis morborum* 6 (ed. Kühn, 7:26).

49. Galen, *De causis morborum* 6 (ed. Kühn, 7:26).

50. Galen, *De naturalibus facultatibus* 3.12–13 (ed. Kühn, 2:185–86; trans. Brock, 286–91).

51. Galen, *De probis malisque alimentorum sucis* 14 (ed. Kühn, 6:814).

52. *Al-waram al-sāʿī:* a translation of the Greek ἕρπης. Ibid.

53. Greek λέπραι. Ibid.

54. Greek ψῶραι. Ibid.

55. Greek κακόχροιαι. Ibid.

56. Galen, *De probis malisque alimentorum sucis* 14 (ed. Kühn, 6:814–15).

57. See introduction, p. xxi.

58. Galen, *In Hippocratis Aphorismos commentarius* 1.2 (ed. Kühn, 17B:359). Compare Anastassiou and Irmer, eds., *Testimonien zum Corpus Hippocraticum,* 307–8.

59. Cf. Strohmaier edition: "Wenn hingegen das Phlegma von übermäßiger, starker und verbrennender Hitze umgeben ist, so kann aus ihm als einzigem von allen Säften keine schwarze Galle entstehen." Galen's commentary on this treatise by Hippocrates only survives in this Arabic translation. I thank Professor Strohmaier for providing me with photocopies of the passages from the forthcoming edition. This quotation does not feature in the Hebrew translation *Airs, Waters, Places,* ed. and trans. Wasserstein.

60. Galen, *De usu partium* 5.6 (ed. Helmreich, 1:270; trans. May, 1:259).

61. Galen, *De naturalibus facultatibus* 2.9 (ed. Kühn, 2:137; trans. Brock, 212–13).

The Third Treatise

1. Galen, *In Hippocratis De natura hominis commentarius tertius* 3.7 (ed. Mewaldt, 95 lines 12–13).

2. Galen, *In Hippocratis Aphorismos commentarius* 5.7 (ed. Kühn, 17B:792), speaks about the age between fourteen and twenty-five as the time of ἥβα (youth, puberty).

3. *Kuhūl:* reflects the Greek παρακμάζω. Galen, *De marcore* 4 (ed. Kühn, 7:680).

4. Greek ὅροι δὲ σαφεῖς. Galen, *De marcore* 4 (ed. Kühn, 7:680).

5. Galen, *De marcore* 4 (ed. Kühn, 7:679–80). The opinion that old age is characterized by coldness and moisture is actually not that of Galen but of his opponents, with whom Galen was engaged in a polemic. Galen himself thought that the temperament of both those past their prime and old people is cold and dry, as stated in the first part of this passage. Cf. Niebyl, "Old Age, Fever, and the Lamp Metaphor," 351–68. For a translation of *De marcore,* see Theoharides, "Galen on Marasmus."

6. "And, since her skin is thick and firm, hardly anything is dissolved through it": cf. Galen, *De causis pulsum* 3.2 (ed. Kühn, 9:111): πυκνόν τε καὶ δύσπνουν τὸ σῶμα.

7. Galen, *De causis pulsum* 3.2 (ed. Kühn, 9:111).

8. Greek οὐ μικρὸν ἀγαθὸν. Galen, *De praesagitione ex pulsibus* 4.4 (ed. Kühn, 9:284).

9. Galen, *De praesagitione ex pulsibus* 4.4 (ed. Kühn, 9:284).

10. Galen, *De optima corporis nostri constitutione* 4 (ed. Kühn, 4:746).

11. "With a loose texture": Greek ἀραιὰ. Galen, *In Hippocratis De alimento commentarius* 4.2 (ed. Kühn, 15:377).

12. "Dense": Greek πυκνὰ. Galen, *In Hippocratis De alimento commentarius* 4.2 (ed. Kühn, 15:377).

13. Galen, *In Hippocratis De alimento commentarius* 4.2 (ed. Kühn, 15:377).

14. The Arabic term *waram* (tumor or swelling) as it appears in the Arabic translations of Galenic texts and in medieval Arabic medical literature is a rather indefinite and vague term, referring to different kinds of tumors and inflammations. Thus, it mostly corresponds to Greek ἱεγμονῆ, i.e., an inflamed swelling or an inflammation. In a few cases we find a more specific term to indicate this specific affliction, namely, *waram ḥārr* (hot tumor). *Waram* can also refer to Greek οἴδημα, i.e., a soft swelling, and to ὄγκος, a "tumor" or "swelling." This vagueness of terminology is reflected in my translation of *waram* as "tumor" or "swelling."

15. Galen, *De curandi ratione per venae sectionem* 7 (ed. Kühn, 11:273). See also Steinschneider, "Griechischen Ärzte," 289 (341), no. 45; *Ḥunain ibn Isḥāq,* ed. and trans. Bergsträsser, no. 71d.

16. Galen, *De plenitudine* 10 (ed. Kühn, 7:562).

17. "The body of the nerves": Greek τοῦ νευρώδους γένους. Galen, *In Hippocratis Epidemiarum I et II* (ed. Wenkebach and Pfaff, 61 line 14).

18. Cf. ibid., 61 lines 13–16; trans. Deller, 521–22, no. 6.

19. Galen, *De curandi ratione per venae sectionem* 9 (ed. Kühn, 11:279).

20. Galen, *De sanitate tuenda* 6.3 (ed. Koch, 176 lines 13–25; trans. Green, 245).

21. Literally, "from the very beginning of the matter"; cf. Greek ἐξ ἀρχῆς.

22. Galen, *De sanitate tuenda* 6.4 (ed. Koch, 176 line 30–177 line 3; trans. Green, 246).

23. **B** reads "wound."

24. "Wound": cf. Galen, *De methodo medendi* 6.2 (ed. Kühn, 10:387): τραύμα.

25. "Allay the pain" *(al-baʿīda ʿan ʾan tūjiʿa):* a translation of the Greek ἀνώδυνον. Galen, *De methodo medendi* 6.2 (ed. Kühn, 10:387). Endress and Gutas, *A Greek and Arabic Lexicon,* 3:306 n. 4, give a variant translation: *taskīn al-ʾalam.*

26. Galen, *De methodo medendi* 6.2 (ed. Kühn, 10:387).

27. Galen, *De methodo medendi* 7.6 (ed. Kühn, 10:495).

28. Galen, *De methodo medendi* 7.7 (ed. Kühn, 10:496), reads τῶν στερεῶν σωμάτων (of the solid organs).

29. Galen, *De methodo medendi* 7.7 (ed. Kühn, 10:496).

30. Cf. Strohmaier edition, 1.8.12 (lines 02911, 02912): "Die Überschüsse der Körper sind im Winter gering, weil die Kälte sie verfestigt, und im Sommer viel, weil die Wärme sie zum Schmelzen bringt." This quotation does not feature in the Hebrew translation edited by Wasserstein.

31. Cf. Strohmaier edition, 1.8.10 (lines 02815, 02816): "Es gibt wenig Leute die zugleich viel essen und trinken können." This quotation does not feature in the Hebrew translation edited by Wasserstein.

32. Cf. Strohmaier edition, 4.5.15 (lines 14803–14807): "Der Samen und das Blut sind nämlich im Winter von einer Art und im Sommer von einer anderen Art. Die Embryos, die in diesen Jahreszeiten entstehen, sind verschieden. So sagen wir jetzt daß Hippokrates die Kälte gemeint hat, also er uns belehren wollte, daß die Mischung des Landes in allen Jahreszeiten eine einzige ist, und als er sagte daß die Kinder einander ähnlich sind. Bei ihnen gibt es nämlich im Sommer keine übermäßige Hitze, welche den Samen verbrennt und austrocknet, und im Winter keine übermäßige Kälte, welche den Samen verfestigt." This quotation does not feature in the Hebrew translation edited by Wasserstein.

33. Strictly speaking, Maimonides is referring to Spica Virginis, a star in the constellation Virgo.

34. Cf. Strohmaier edition, 2.5.3 (lines 08801–08804): "So wäre es für Hippokrates angemessener gewesen für die Jahreszeiten und Zeiträume Grenzen und Abschnitte festzulegen und sie so deutlicher zu machen und zu sagen, daß die Tagundnachtgleiche nach dem Winter der Beginn des Frühjahrs ist und daß der Aufgang der Plejaden der Beginn des Sommers und ihr Untergang des Winters ist. Wenn er also die Tagundnachtgleiche nach dem Sommer nicht als Anfang des Herbstes ansetzen und festlegen wollte, so hätte er doch sagen können, daß der Aufgang des Arkturos der Anfang des Herbstes ist"; see as well *Airs, Waters, Places,* ed. and trans. Wasserstein, 84–87 (268–71).

35. "Vessels", i.e., veins, cf. Galen.

36. "In wounds"; cf. Galen, *De semine* 1.13 (Galen, *On Semen,* ed. and trans. Phillip de Lacy, 110 line 1): ἐν ἕλκεσι.

37. "Quite important and marvelous" *(sāliḥa fī al-ʿiẓam wa-fī al-ʿadad):* reflects the Greek ἱκανῶς ἀξιολόγους τε καὶ πολλάς. Galen, *De semine* 1.13 (Galen, *On Semen,* ed. and trans. de Lacy, 110 line 2).

38. Galen, *De semine* 1.13 (Galen, *On Semen,* ed. and trans. de Lacy, 110 lines 3–4), reads οὔτε πολλοῖς φθησαν ἐν ἕλκεσι γεννηθεῖσαι ἱέβες (veins generated in wounds have not been seen by many persons but by very few).

39. Galen, *De semine* 1.13 (Galen, *On Semen,* ed. and trans. de Lacy, 108 line 27–110 line 6).

40. Galen, *De arte parva* 16 (ed. Kühn, 1:347; ed. Boudon, 323–24). Véronique Boudon does not deal with Maimonides' quotations from this treatise in her admirable edition.

41. Galen, *De usu partium* 13.8 (ed. Helmreich, 2:262, 264; trans. May, 2:603, 605).

42. "Part of it is connected to the members of hands and feet through its fleshy parts": cf. Galen, *De usu partium* 12.2 (ed. Helmreich, 2:188). Trans. May, 2:553, reads "which becomes soft bedding for the animal when it falls or lies down."

43. Galen, *De usu partium* 12.2 (ed. Helmreich, 2:188; trans. May, 2:553).

44. Meaning "in order of use"; cf. the Galenic continuation of this passage. Here I am following May.

45. Galen, *De usu partium* 11.11 (ed. Helmreich, 2:147–48; trans. May, 2:526).

46. "On both sides": Galen, *De usu partium* 14.14 (ed. Helmreich, 2:334 lines 5–6), reads καὶ τἆλλα τὰ περικείμενα. Trans. May, 2:653, renders this as "and other surrounding parts." See also **E**.

47. Galen, *De usu partium* 14.14 (ed. Helmreich, 2:334; trans. May, 2:653).

48. "Affected by": Galen, *De methodo medendi* 6.3 (ed. Kühn, 10:403), reads βλάπτεται (harmed by).

49. Galen, *De methodo medendi* 6.3 (ed. Kühn, 10:403).

50. Cf. Strohmaier edition, 1.10.1 (lines 03809–03813): "Jede Stadt die in Richtung des Sonnenuntergangs liegt, ist gegen die Ostwinde geschützt. Zu ihr wehen die warmen Winde und die kalten aus der Richting der beiden Kälber. So ist diese Stadt unweigerlich schlecht, verpestet und voll von Krankheiten. Galen sagt: Als Hippokrates diese Stadt und ihre Lage erwähnte, hat er uns mit seinen Worten darauf hingewiesen, daß sie die schlechteste aller Städte ist, wegen der Verschiedenheit ihrer Luft. . . ." *Airs, Waters, Places,* ed. and trans. Wasserstein, 40–41 (224–25).

51. Cf. Galen, *De symptomatum causis* 3.1, 3 (ed. Kühn, 7:213, 221).

52. That is, anasarca (ἀνά σάρκα).

53. Galen, *De inaequali intemperie* 1 (ed. Kühn, 7:733).

54. "Which diminishes his strength": Galen, *In Hippocratis Epidemiarum* 6.1–8 (ed. Wenkebach and Pfaff, 232 line 9), has καταλύεται μὲν ἡ δύναμις. Trans. Deller, 537, no. 82, reads "durch die Schwäche der Kraft."

55. Galen, *In Hippocratis Epidemiarum* 6.1–8 (ed. Wenkebach and Pfaff, 232 lines 4–12).

56. "Animal faculty," i.e., vital faculty. The Greek term ζωτικός, especially in combination with πνεῦμα, has become in Arabic, as a result of a wrong translation, *ḥayawānī* (animal); see Ullmann, *Medizin im Islam,* 63.

57. Galen, *De praesagitione ex pulsibus* 4.11 (ed. Kühn, 9:420), reads οἷον πνίξεις (is as it were strangulated).

58. Galen, *De praesagitione ex pulsibus* 4.11 (ed. Kühn, 9:419–20).

59. Galen, *De methodo medendi* 11.3 (ed. Kühn, 10:742), mentions τῶν στερεῶν (the solid parts [of the body]). The Arabic *al-aṣlīya* (main) is possibly a corruption of *al-ṣaliba* (solid).

60. Galen, *De methodo medendi* 11.3 (ed. Kühn, 10:742), speaks about the vapor arising from the blood (τοῦ αἵματος ἀναθυμιάσεως).

61. Galen, *De methodo medendi* 11.3 (ed. Kühn, 10:742), has τῶν στερεῶν (solid parts). Cf. n. 59 of this treatise.

62. Galen, *De methodo medendi* 11.3 (ed. Kühn, 10:742).

63. Galen, *In Hippocratis Aphorismos commentarius* 2.47 (ed. Kühn, 17B:550–51).

64. Galen, *De marcore* 5 (ed. Kühn, 7:683). For an English translation, see Theoharides, trans., "Galen on Marasmus," 369–90.

65. Galen, *De naturalibus facultatibus* 3.13 (ed. Kühn 2:189–90; trans. Brock, 292–95).

66. Galen, *De usu partium* 4.4–6 (ed. Helmreich, 1:199–200; trans. May, 1:206–7).

67. That is, it is filled with *pneuma*, or "vital spirit," inhaled from the air.

68. Galen, *De usu partium* 4.15 (ed. Helmreich, 1:235; trans. May, 1:234).

69. Galen, *De usu partium* 4.17–18 (ed. Helmreich, 1:239–42; trans. May, 1:237–38).

70. Galen, *De usu partium* 5.6–7 (ed. Helmreich, 1:272–73; trans. May, 1:260–61).

71. "[There] and by the length of the distance [it covers]": Galen, *De usu partium* 7.22 (ed. Helmreich, 1:439) reads ἀεικινήτῳ μορίῳ. Trans. May, 1:381, has "in a part that is always in motion."

72. Galen, *De usu partium* 7.22 (ed. Helmreich, 1:439; trans. May, 1:381).

73. Galen, *De usu partium* 14.7 (ed. Helmreich, 2:307; trans. May, 2:636).

74. Galen, *De usu partium* 14.8 (ed. Helmreich, 2:310; trans. May, 2:638).

75. Galen, *De symptomatum causis* 1.7 (ed. Kühn, 7:130), has συμπτώματα (symptoms).

76. Or "vital desire," or "spiritual desire." Galen, *De symptomatum causis* 1.7 (ed. Kühn, 7:131), reads ἡ ὄρεξις αὐτῆς ἡ ψυχικὴ ἁπασῶν ὑστάτη.

77. Galen, *De symptomatum causis* 1.7 (ed. Kühn, 7:130–31).

78. *Nafkha:* Blowing or other forceful exhalation; it is a translation of the Greek ἐκφυσήσις. Galen, *De locis affectis* 4.9 (ed. Kühn, 8:270).

79. Galen, *De locis affectis* 4.9 (ed. Kühn, 8:270); trans. Siegel, 125.

80. "Noiseless exsufflation": Galen, *De locis affectis* 4.9 (ed. Kühn, 8:270), reads ψοφώδη (noisy exsufflation). Galen's version also features in MS Wellcome Or. 14a.

81. "Uvula, and upper palate": translated according to **ESGLBP** and MS Wellcome Or. 14a to read "upper parts of the uvula and palate."

82. Galen, *De locis affectis* 4.9 (ed. Kühn, 8:271–72; trans. Siegel, 126).

83. Literally, "escapes nature so that it cannot turn it."

84. Galen, *In Hippocratis Prognostica commentarius* 1.42 (ed. Kühn, 18B:109), reads οὔθ' ὡς τὸ αἷμα μεταβληθὲν ὑπ' αὐτῆς (It is not like the blood changed by it).

85. The Arabic text seems to be corrupt. A possible emendation is ولا هو بمنزلة المدّة التي تفعلها وأحالتها الطبيعة في الحال الخارجة عن الطبع (and it is not like pus, which is generated and changed by [nature] in unnatural conditions). Cf. Galen, *In Hippocratis Prognostica commentaries* 1.42 (ed. Kühn, 18B:109): οὔθ' ὡς τὸ πῦον τῆς παρὰ φύσιν αἰτιάς ἐν τῇ γενέσει μεταλαβόν (nor like the pus changed in the generation because of a cause which is contrary to nature).

86. Galen, *In Hippocratis Prognostica commentarius* 2.38–39 (ed. Kühn, 18B:165–68).
87. See 2.17 of translated text, p. 31.
88. "Is corrupted": Galen, *De curandi ratione per venae sectionem* 5 (ed. Kühn, 11:262), reads ἐλάττων (becomes less).
89. Galen, *De curandi ratione per venae sectionem* 5 (ed. Kühn, 11:262).
90. Galen, *De usu partium* 9.4 (ed. Helmreich, 2:13–14; trans. May, 1:433).
91. In effect, "is loose"; see Galen, *De tumoribus praeter naturam* 2 (ed. Kühn, 7:714), χαλαρόν.
92. *Mawāḍi*[c]: Literally, "places." This is a translation of the Greek χῶραι (Galen, *De tum. praet. nat.* 2 [ed. Kühn, 7:714]), which in general means "places" but also "spaces."
93. That is, diastole.
94. Galen, *De tum. praet. nat.* 2 (ed. Kühn, 7:714).
95. Galen, *In Hippocratis Epidemiarum* 6.1–8 (ed. Wenkebach and Pfaff, 239 lines 1–4, 21–22); trans. Deller, 537, no. 83. See also Anastassiou and Irmer, *Testimonien zum Corpus Hippokraticum,* 67.
96. Galen, *De atra bile* 7 (ed. Kühn, 5:136; ed. de Boer, 136).
97. Galen, *De methodo medendi* 14.6 (ed. Kühn, 10:963), reads "Inflations originate from flatuous winds."
98. Galen, *De methodo medendi* 14.6 (ed. Kühn, 10:963).
99. That is, passage of the nourishment through a membrane or other permeable substance. The literal translation is "sweating through"; see the Greek: διάδοσις. Galen, *De usu partium* 10.1 (ed. Helmreich, 2:56). An important and controversial example from Galenic physiology concerned the supposed transudation of blood from the right to the left cardiac ventricles through the supposedly porous intraventricular septum.
100. Galen, *De usu partium* 10.1 (ed. Helmreich, 2:56; trans. May, 2:464–65).
101. Galen, *De usu partium* 13.9 (ed. Helmreich, 2:265; trans. May, 2:605).
102. Galen, *De usu partium* 16.2 (ed. Helmreich, 2:381; trans. May, 2:684). See also trans. Savage-Smith, 60–61 (Arabic), 114 (English).
103. "Many nerves . . . not need sensation": This sentence seems to be a summary of Galen, *De usu partium* 16.3 (ed. Helmreich, 2:282; trans. May, 2:685); see also trans. Savage-Smith, 62 (Arabic), 116 (English).
104. Galen, *De usu partium* 16.2 (ed. Helmreich, 2:382; trans. May, 2:685); see also trans. Savage-Smith, 61 (Arabic), 115 (English). This text recurs in Maimonides, *Medical Aphorisms* 25.36 (ed. Bos).
105. Literally, "Just as sensation includes the skin."
106. Galen, *De usu partium* 16.2 (ed. Helmreich, 2:380; trans. May, 2:684). See also trans. Savage-Smith, 60 (Arabic), 113–14 (English).
107. Galen, *De symptomatum causis* 1.5 (ed. Kühn, 7:113–14).
108. Added according to Galen, *De symptomatum causis* 2.2 (ed. Kühn, 7:160): οὐ γὰρ δὴ τά γε ὀστᾶ καὶ οἱ χόνδροι πάλλονταί ποτε.
109. Galen, *De symptomatum causis* 2.2 (ed. Kühn, 7:159–60); cf. n. 106 in treatise 1.

110. Galen, *De curandi ratione per venae sectionem* 8 (ed. Kühn, 11:275) reads οἱ ἀδένες καὶ αἱ σάρκες (glands and [other kinds of] flesh).

111. Galen, *De curandi ratione per venae sectionem* 8 (ed. Kühn, 11:275).

112. Pseudo-Galen, *In Hippocratis De alimento commentarius* 1 (ed. Kühn, 15:224–28); the quotation does not appear in this fragmentary section of Galen's commentary.

113. This treatise of Galen's, *De somno et vigilia,* survives only in an Arabic translation. See Nabielek, trans., "'Über Schlaf und Wachsein.'" For Maimonides' quotation, see pp. 35–36. Cf. Strohmaier, "Der syrische und arabische Galen," 2015, no. 13.

114. Galen, *De differentiis febrium* 1.7 (ed. Kühn, 7:299–300).

115. Galen, *De naturalibus facultatibus* 3.13 (ed. Kühn 2:187–94; trans. Brock, 290–301).

116. Galen, *Ad Glauconem de methodo medendi* 2.9 (ed. Kühn, 11:116).

117. Galen, *De usu partium* 14.13 (ed. Helmreich, 2:331–32; trans. May, 2:651).

118. Galen, *In Hippocratis Prognostica commentarius* 1.42 (ed. Kühn, 18B:107), reads: τοῦτο γοῦν τὸ αἷμα κατὰ μικρὰ μέρια παρεσπαρμένον τοῖς ἱεγμαίνουσι μορίοις . . . ἐπανελθεῖν μὲν εἰς τὴν ἀρχαίαν φύσιν οὐκέτι δύναται. μεταβάλλεται δὲ καὶ σῦπεται. . . . ἐὰν μὲν οὖν ἐπὶ πλεῖστον ᾖ ἐξεστηκὸς τῆς οἰκείας εὐκρασίας τὸ ἔμφυτον θερμὸν, ὡς ἐν ἀψύχῳ σώματι σῦπεται τὸ αἷμα (When that blood that is in the organs that are afflicted with a tumor is diffused in small parts . . . it cannot return to its former nature. It is transformed and putrefies. . . . When the innate heat departs from its proper balance, the blood putrefies, as in a dead body).

119. Galen, *In Hippocratis Prognostica commentarius* 1.42 (ed. Kühn, 18B:107–8).

120. Galen, *De inaequali intemperie* 3 (ed. Kühn, 7:736–37).

121. Galen, *In Hipp. Epid. 1 & 2,* 173 line 24–174 line 14); trans. Deller, 531, no. 52.

122. *Fālij:* See Richter-Bernburg, trans., "De Theriaca ad Pisonem," 204.

123. Galen, *In Hippocratis Epidemiarum* 6.1–8 (ed. Wenkebach and Pfaff, 387 lines 30–39; 388 lines 9–10); trans. Deller, 541–42, no. 105.

124. This quotation is possibly an adaptation of Galen, *De methodo medendi* 7.7 (ed. Kühn, 10:500).

125. Cf. Galen, *De differentiis febrium* 1.6 (ed. Kühn, 7:290–91): ἡ τοῦ μέλλοντος πάσχειν σώματος ἑτοιμότης.

126. Galen, *De differentiis febrium* 1.6 (ed. Kühn, 7:290–91).

127. "Change in weather": Galen, *De pulsibus libellus ad tirones* 9 (ed. Kühn, 8:470), has καταστάσεις ἀέρος (the [different] conditions of the weather); for the Arabic name of this treatise, see Ullmann, *Medizin im Islam,* 44, no. 32.

128. Galen, *De pulsibus libellus ad tirones* 11 (ed. Kühn, 8:470).

129. Galen, *De praesagitione ex pulsibus* 2.4 (ed. Kühn, 9:283).

130. Galen, *De sanitate tuenda* 5.4 (ed. Koch, 143 lines 10–16; trans. Green, 201–2).

131. Galen, *De sanitate tuenda* 1.4 (ed. Koch, 6 line 33–7 line 7; trans. Green, 11).

132. Galen, *De sanitate tuenda* 6.5–6 (ed. Koch, 179 lines 12–17; trans. Green, 250).

133. Galen, *De sanitate tuenda* 6.6 (ed. Koch, 179 lines 15–21, 180 lines 19–20; trans. Green, 251–52).

134. Cf. Galen, *In Hippocratis De alimento commentarius* 4 (ed. Kühn, 15:415): προστίθησί τι.

135. Galen, *In Hippocratis De alimento commentarius* 4 (ed. Kühn, 15:415).

136. Literally, "hemorrhoids."

137. See introduction, p. xxi, and introduction, n. 34.

138. *Waswās:* Greek παραφροσύνας. Galen, *De usu partium* 11.3 (ed. Helmreich, 2:118 line 5). Cf. 2.16 of translated text, p. 31.

139. Galen, *De usu partium* 11.3 (ed. Helmreich, 2:118; trans. May, 2:507).

140. Galen, *De symptomatum causis* 1.2 (ed. Kühn, 7:94).

141. Galen, *In Hippocratis Prognostica commentarius* 1.30 (ed. Kühn, 18B:92–93).

142. Galen refers to inspiration and expiration through the whole body: ἥ τε ἀναπνοὴ καὶ ἡ καθ' ὅλον τὸ σῶμα διαπνοή. Galen, *In Hipp. Epid.* 6, 258 lines 18–19.

143. *In Hipp. Epid.* 6, 258 lines 13–19.

144. Galen, *De sanitate tuenda* 6.10 (ed. Koch, 187 line 31), reads χαλεπὴ δὲ γίνεται μίξις (and a troublesome combination occurs); see also trans. Green, 263.

145. Galen, *De sanitate tuenda* 6.10 (ed. Koch, 188 lines 1–2; trans. Green, 263) reads χειρίστη δέ ὅταν οὕτως ἔχῃ κατασκευῆς τε καὶ φύσεως ὁ ἄνθρωπος ὡς μήτ' εὔλυτον ἔχειν γαστέρα μήτ' ἐμεῖν ἑτοίμως (but the worst is when the patient is of such a constitution and nature that he has a stomach neither easy to purge nor ready to vomit).

146. Galen, *De sanitate tuenda* 6.10 (ed. Koch, 187 line 31–188 line 2; trans. Green, 263).

147. Galen, *De methodo medendi* 12.8 (ed. Kühn, 10:872), reads ταῖς ὀλεθρίαις φρενίτισι (with deadly inflammations of the brain).

148. Galen, *De methodo medendi* 12.8 (ed. Kühn, 10:872).

149. "Something similar . . . the nerves" *(shabīh bi al-jumūd fī al-aʿṣāb).* This reflects the Greek: ὅμοιον τι πήξει (Galen, *De methodo medendi* 12.8 [ed. Kühn, 10:872]).

150. Galen, *De methodo medendi* 12.8 (ed. Kühn, 10:872).

151. Galen, *De compositione medicamentorum secundum locos* 2.1 (ed. Kühn, 12:499–500); cf. n. 33 of treatise 2, above.

152. Galen, *De compositione medicamentorum secundum locos* 3.2 (ed. Kühn, 12:664), reads παρωτίδες (inflammations of the parotid glands).

153. Galen, *De compositione medicamentorum secundum locos* 3.2 (ed. Kühn, 12:664–65).

154. "Abscesses occurring in the roots of ears": cf. n. 152 of this treatise.

155. Galen, *De compositione medicamentorum secundum locos* 3.2 (ed. Kühn, 12:665).

156. Galen, *De compositione medicamentorum secundum locos* 4.1 (ed. Kühn, 12:706).

157. Galen, *De praesagitione ex pulsibus* 4.4 (ed. Kühn, 9:399), reads ἀλλὰ καὶ τῇ συμφύτῳ δυνάμει ῥᾳδίως ἀλλοιοῖ τὸ ἱέγμα (but also because of its innate faculty it easily transforms the phlegm).

158. Galen, *De praesagitione ex pulsibus* 4.4 (ed. Kühn, 9:399–400).

159. Galen, *De methodo medendi* 11.15 (ed. Kühn, 10:787), reads μάλιστα δ' ὅταν εἰς ἧπαρ ἢ γαστέρα κατασκήπτῃ τὰ περιττὰ τοῖς στύφουσι χρῆσθαι· κύριά τε γὰρ ἱκανῶς τὰ μόρια καὶ πάντως ἐργάζεσθαι τὸ σφέτερον ἔργον ἀναγκαῖα κᾀν ταῖς νόσοις (Astringent drugs should be used above all when superfluities stream to the liver or stomach. For these organs are so important that they also have to carry out their own task during illnesses).

160. Galen, *De methodo medendi* 11.15 (ed. Kühn, 10:787, 794).

161. Maimonides' discussion is probably based on Galen, *De methodo medendi* 13.5 (ed. Kühn, 10:881).

162. Literally, "cannot be resolved"; cf. Galen, *De methodo medendi* 13.15 (ed. Kühn, 10:917): ἀλύτους.

163. Galen, *De methodo medendi* 13.15 (ed. Kühn, 10:914, 917).

164. Literally, "hard tumors"; cf. Galen, *De methodo medendi* 13.15 (ed. Kühn, 10:917): αἱ σκιρρώδεις διαθέσεις.

165. Galen, *De methodo medendi* 13.15 (ed. Kühn, 10:914, 917).

166. Cf. Galen, *De methodo medendi* 6.4 (ed. Kühn, 10:419): τὸ λεπτὸν καὶ νευρῶδες τοῦ χιτῶνος.

167. Cf. Galen, *De methodo medendi* 6.4 (ed. Kühn, 10:419).

168. Greek: ἐπιδερμὶς. Galen, *De simplicium medicamentorum temperamentis ac facultatibus* 11.1 (ed. Kühn, 12:319).

169. Cf. Galen, *De simplicium medicamentorum temperamentis ac facultatibus* 11.1 (ed. Kühn, 12:319): αἱ λέπραι (see 2.16 of translated text, p. 31 and n. 37 of treatise 2).

170. Galen, *De simplicium medicamentorum temperamentis ac facultatibus* 11.1 (ed. Kühn, 12:319–20).

171. Galen, *De pulsibus libellus ad tirones* 12 (ed. Kühn, 8:479–80).

172. Greek: ἐκπυήσις. Galen, *In Hippocratis Prognostica commentarius* 1.35 (ed. Kühn, 18B:98).

173. Literally, "is delayed for twenty days."

174. According to Galen, *In Hippocratis Prognostica commentarius* 1.35 (ed. Kühn, 18B:98), suppuration occurs in tumors if the fever does not abate after the twentieth day, and in cold tumors, after the sixtieth day.

175. Galen, *In Hippocratis Prognostica commentarius* 1.35 (ed. Kühn, 18B:98).

176. Galen, *De locis affectis* 5.2 (ed. Kühn, 8:303; trans. Siegel, 138).

177. Galen, *De praes. ex pulsu* 4.1, 3–5 (ed. Kühn, 9:392, 399–400).

178. Takhalkhul: Greek ἀραιότης. Galen, *In Hippocratis Prognostica commentarius* 2.68 (ed. Kühn, 18B:219).

179. Galen, *In Hippocratis Prognostica commentarius* 2.68 (ed. Kühn, 18B:219).

180. Galen, *De crisibus* 3.7 (ed. Kühn, 9:33).

181. Galen, *De crisibus* 3.9 (ed. Kühn, 9:742).

182. Galen, *De crisibus* 3.11 (ed. Kühn, 9:759–68).

183. Galen, *De crisibus* 3.9 (ed. Kühn, 9:745).

184. Literally, "things."

185. Literally, "moistures."

186. Galen, *De locis affectis* 6.6 (ed. Kühn, 8:439; trans. Siegel, 192–93).

187. Galen, *De methodo medendi* 13.4, 6 (ed. Kühn, 10:893, 903–4).
188. Galen, *De methodo medendi* 13.19 (ed. Kühn, 10:925).
189. Galen, *De methodo medendi* 13.19 (ed. Kühn, 10:926).
190. Galen, *De methodo medendi* 13.22 (ed. Kühn, 10:938–39).
191. Galen, *De compositione medicamentorum secundum locos* 5.5 (ed. Kühn, 12:854).
192. Galen, *De methodo medendi* 14.3 (ed. Kühn, 10:950).
193. Galen, *De compositione medicamentorum secundum locos* 7.2 (ed. Kühn, 13:25).
194. Galen, *De methodo medendi* 12.6 (ed. Kühn, 10:846).
195. Galen, *De compositione medicamentorum per genera* 3.3 (ed. Kühn, 13:614); for the title *Qaṭājānas,* see Ullmann, *Medizin im Islam,* 48–49, no. 50.
196. Galen, *In Hippocratis Aphorismos commentarius* 1.15 (ed. Kühn, 17B:421); the statement is quoted by Galen in the name of Diocles.

The Fourth Treatise

1. Galen, *De praesagitione ex pulsibus* 1.1 (ed. Kühn, 9:210), refers to the generation of the psychical pneuma (γένεσις πνεύματος ψυχικοῦ).
2. Galen, *De praesagitione ex pulsibus* 1.1 (ed. Kühn, 9:210).
3. *Wazn:* "Weight" or "measure"; it is used to translate the Greek ῥυθμὸς. Galen, *De differentia pulumm* 1.6; (ed. Kühn, 8:512).
4. This seems to mean that sometimes the person will have a pulse rhythm that sounds like that of other men his age and sometimes it will be different, perhaps because he has been exercising. Or it may mean that some men will have a pulse rhythm that sounds like that of other men their age but that the pulse of others will differ because they are in a different state of health or fitness.
5. Galen, *De differentia pulumm* 1.6; (ed. Kühn, 8:512).
6. "Far from correctly" *(ba^cīdan ^can al-ḥaqīqī).* In the Greek it is πόρρω τῆς ἀκριβοῦς (far from exact). Galen, *De differentia pulumm* 7.3 (ed. Kühn, 8:907).
7. Galen, *De differentia pulumm* 7.3 (ed. Kühn, 8:907).
8. In this section on the pulse, "the faculty," when named without any further definition, refers to the animal faculty. On the pulse, cf. Adams. trans., *The Seven Books of Paulus Aegineta* 1.12 (1:214–15): "According to Galen, the pulse consists of four parts: of a diastole and a systole with two intervals of rest, one after the diastole before the systole, and the other after the systole before the diastole. The first distinctions of the pulse are derived from the extent of the diastole, according to its three dimensions, namely, length, breadth, and depth. These give rise to the characters *long, broad,* and *deep* or *high.* The characters of *quick* (rapid) and *slow* are derived from the length of time occupied in the actions of systole and diastole. The distinctions of *strong* and *feeble* (weak) are derived from the force with which the artery strikes the finger. The relaxation and constriction of the arterial tube give rise to the characters of *soft* and *hard.* The characters of *dense* and *rare* are derived from the time which elapses between two diastoles or pulsations of the artery. The

terms *equal* and *unequal* arise from the constancy or inconstancy of any peculiar character of the arterial pulsation. The *regular* and *irregular* are distinguished from these, inasmuch as a series of pulsations, although unequal may be regular, when they observe a certain ratio."

The Arabic term translated as "strong" refers to forcefulness; the term translated as "great" indicates extent or magnitude. Hence, Maimonides interprets a strong pulse as one whose beat is distinctly felt and a great pulse as one that is apparent throughout the body.

9. Galen, *De curandi ratione per venae sectionem* 13 (ed. Kühn, 11:291).

10. "Extremely slow and rare" *(fī ghāya al-tafāwut):* in the Greek it is ἀραιότατος. Galen, *De causis pulsum* 11.5 (ed. Kühn, 9:118).

11. Galen, *De causis pulsum* 11.5 (ed. Kühn, 9:118–19).

12. Galen, *De praesagitione ex pulsibus* 2.5 (ed. Kühn, 9:291).

13. "Inequality" *(ikhtilāf)* is a translation of the Greek ἀνωμαλία. Galen, *De praesagitione ex pulsibus* 2.13 (ed. Kühn, 9:328).

14. Galen, *De praesagitione ex pulsibus* 2.13 (ed. Kühn, 9:328).

15. Galen, *De causis pulsum* 2.14 (ed. Kühn, 9:102).

16. That is, artery.

17. Galen, *De causis pulsum* 2.1 (ed. Kühn, 9:56).

18. Galen, *De causis pulsum* 2.1 (ed. Kühn, 9:59–60).

19. Galen, *De causis pulsum* 2.3 (ed. Kühn, 9:65), reads παλινδρομοῦντας.

20. "It turns one's pulse into the recurrent one called 'mouse tail'" *(wa-taj*ʿ*al al-nabḍ al-musammā dhanab al-fa*ʾ*r);* this is a translation of the Greek τῶν μυούρων ἐστὶ σφυγμῶν ἀποτελεστική. Galen, *De causis pulsum* 2.3 (ed. Kühn, 9:65).

21. Galen, *De causis pulsum* 2.3 (ed. Kühn, 9:65).

22. "The vibratory and spasmodic pulses": Greek ὅ τε κλονώδης καὶ ὅ σπασμώδης. Galen, *De dignoscendis pulsibus* 4.1 (ed. Kühn, 8:922).

23. Galen, *De dignoscendis pulsibus* 4.1 (ed. Kühn, 8:922).

24. Galen, *De dignoscendis pulsibus* 1.5 (ed. Kühn, 8:795–96).

25. Cf. Galen, *De dignoscendis pulsibus* 1.5 (ed. Kühn, 8:795): ὅστις γὰρ ἂν μέγιστός θ' ἅμα καὶ σφοδρότατος καὶ σκληρὸς, καθ' ὅσον οἷόν τε μεγέθει μιχθῆναι σκληρότητα, καὶ μὴ ταχὺς, σαφεστάτην οὗτος ἔχει τὴν συστολήν (For the pulse that is very great and at the same time very strong and hard, and to the same extent the pulse that combines greatness with hardness without rapidity, has the clearest contraction).

26. Galen, *De dignoscendis pulsibus* 1.5, 9 (ed. Kühn, 8:795, 816).

27. Galen, *De pulsibus libellus ad tirones* 12 (ed. Kühn, 8:490).

28. Galen, *De pulsibus libellus ad tirones* 12 (ed. Kühn, 8:483).

29. Galen, *De pulsibus libellus ad tirones* 10–11 (ed. Kühn, 8:468, 471).

30. "Cooler than its natural temperament": Galen, *De praesagitione ex pulsibus* 3.3 (ed. Kühn, 9:340–41), reads τοῦ σπλάγχνου ψυχρότερόν ἐστι τοῦ κατὰ φύσιν.

31. Galen, *De praesagitione ex pulsibus* 3.3 (ed. Kühn, 9:341), reads διαθέσεις (constitutions or bodily conditions).

32. Galen, *De praesagitione ex pulsibus* 3.3 (ed. Kühn, 9:340–41).

33. Galen, *De differentiis febrium* 1.9 (ed. Kühn, 7:306–7).
34. Galen, *De pulsibus libellus ad tirones* 12 (ed. Kühn, 8:489–90).
35. Galen, *De causis pulsum* 2.6 (ed. Kühn, 9:78), refers to different parts of the artery (διαφέροντα μόρια τῆς ἀρτηρίας).
36. Galen, *De causis pulsum* 2.6 (ed. Kühn, 9:78).
37. Literally, "very far from being untrue."
38. Cf. Galen, *De praesagitione ex pulsibus* 3.5 (ed. Kühn, 9:364): ἐπεὶ κατά γε τὰς ἀκμὰς ἧττον.
39. Cf. Galen, *De praesagitione ex pulsibus* 3.5 (ed. Kühn, 9:374).
40. Galen, *De praesagitione ex pulsibus* 3.7 (ed. Kühn, 9:379–80).
41. "Considerable": the Arabic equivalent is *dhū qadr yuʿtaddu bihi* (literally, "of [such] a size that it is taken into consideration"), which is a translation of the Greek ἀξιόλογος. Galen, *De praesagitione ex pulsibus* 3.7 (ed. Kühn, 9:384).
42. Galen, *De praesagitione ex pulsibus* 3.7 (ed. Kühn, 9:384).
43. Galen remarks that those arteries which are far from the diseased organ or those for whom the heart mediates change less (τὰς δ' ἤτοι πόρρω τῶν πεπονθότων ἢ διὰ μέσης τῆς καρδίας ἧττον). Galen, *De praesagitione ex pulsibus* 4.9 (ed. Kühn, 9:414).
44. Galen, *De praesagitione ex pulsibus* 4.9 (ed. Kühn, 9:414).
45. Galen, *De praesagitione ex pulsibus* 4.12 (ed. Kühn, 9:421).
46. Galen, *De praesagitione ex pulsibus* 1.4 (ed. Kühn, 9:244).
47. Galen, *De praesagitione ex pulsibus* 1.4 (ed. Kühn, 9:245).
48. Galen, *De crisibus* 3.11 (ed. Kühn, 9:764), reads καὶ μάλιστ' ἐπειδὰν ἀγωνιστικόν τι καὶ παρακινδυνευτικὸν ἔχωσι (and especially when these crises come with something of a struggle and danger).
49. "Undulatory" *(mawjī)* is a translation of the Greek κυματώδης. Galen, *De crisibus* 3.11 (ed. Kühn, 9:763).
50. Literally, "blood"; cf. Galen, *De crisibus* 3.11 (ed. Kühn, 9:763): αἱμορραγία.
51. "A high pulse and a strong pulse . . . are both"; cf. Galen, *De crisibus* 3.11 (ed. Kühn, 9:763): ὁ μὲν γὰρ ὑψηλὸς καθάπερ καὶ ὁ σφοδρός.
52. Galen, *De crisibus* 3.11 (ed. Kühn, 9:763–64).
53. Galen, *De causis pulsum* 1.7 (ed. Kühn, 9:23–24).
54. Galen, *De causis pulsum* 2.2 (ed. Kühn, 9:63).
55. Galen, *De causis pulsum* 1.9 (ed. Kühn, 9:37–38).
56. Galen, *De differentia pulumm* 1.26 (ed. Kühn, 8:553).
57. Galen, *De pulsibus libellus ad tirones* 11 (ed. Kühn, 8:473).
58. Galen, *De differentiis febrium* 1.9 (ed. Kühn, 7:311–12).
59. "Of those suffering from spasms" *(aṣḥāb al-tashannuj):* Greek τῶν σπωμένων. Galen, *De pulsibus libellus ad tirones* 12 (ed. Kühn, 8:487).
60. Cf. Galen, *De pulsibus libellus ad tirones* 12 (ed. Kühn, 8:487): διὰ μὲν τὴν τάσιν εὔρωστος φαινομένη.
61. Cf. Galen, *De pulsibus libellus ad tirones* 12 (ed. Kühn, 8:487): διὰ δὲ τὸν κλόνον ἐκπηδητική.
62. Galen, *De pulsibus libellus ad tirones* 12 (ed. Kühn, 8:487).
63. Galen, *De dignoscendis pulsibus* 1.11 (ed. Kühn, 8:819–20).
64. Galen, *De dignoscendis pulsibus* 1.11 (ed. Kühn, 8:821).

65. Cf. Galen, *De causis pulsum* 2.6 (ed. Kühn, 9:76): ὅταν ἡ μὲν δύναμις εὔρωστος ᾖ, τὸ δ' ὄργανον σκληρὸν, ἐπείγῃ δ' ἡ χρεία. For the term "need" *(ḥāja)*, cf. Galen, *On Respiration and the Arteries*, ed. and trans. Furley and Wilkie, 58–60.

66. Galen, *De causis pulsum* 2.6 (ed. Kühn, 9:76).

67. "Dense": cf. Galen, *De praesagitione ex pulsibus* 1.7 (ed. Kühn, 9:266): πυκνὸν. The Arabic *mutawātir* seems to represent both the Greek σπασμώδης (spasmodic) and πυκνὸς (dense).

68. "Very rare"; Cf. Galen, *De praesagitione ex pulsibus* 1.7 (ed. Kühn, 9:266): καὶ ἀραιότερον.

69. Galen, *De praesagitione ex pulsibus* 1.7 (ed. Kühn, 9:266).

70. Meaning the arteries.

71. Galen, *De causis pulsum* 2.8 (ed. Kühn, 9:81).

72. "In many . . . pulses": cf. Galen, *De praesagitione ex pulsibus* 2.4 (ed. Kühn, 9:280): ἐν ἀθροίσματι.

73. Galen, *De praesagitione ex pulsibus* 2.4 (ed. Kühn, 9:279–80).

74. "Dense": cf. Galen, *De praesagitione ex pulsibus* 1.24; (ed. Kühn, 9:201): πυκνότερον.

75. Literally, "hydrops of the flesh."

76. I.e., arteries.

77. Galen, *De causis pulsum* 4.24 (ed. Kühn, 9:202) remarks that anasarca makes the pulse soft, undulatory, and broader (μαλακούς τε καὶ κυματώδεις καὶ πλατυτέρους).

78. Galen, *De causis pulsum* 4.24 (ed. Kühn, 9:201–2).

79. Galen, *De praesagitione ex pulsibus* 4.5 (ed. Kühn, 9:401).

80. Section 43 in Muntner's edition of the Hebrew translation by Nathan ha-Meʾati is identical with section 45 in our edition of the Arabic text. Thus, the same text also features in Muntner's edition as section 45, but with some minor variations. One of the manuscripts consulted by Muntner, i.e., ב, actually has this text only as a marginal gloss.

81. Galen, *De dignoscendis pulsibus* 3.2 (ed. Kühn, 8:888–99).

82. Galen, *De causis pulsum* 1.7 (ed. Kühn, 9:25).

83. That is, dicrotic; the Arabic *dhū al-qarʿatayn* stands for the Greek δίκροτος; Galen, *De causis pulsum* 1.6 (ed. Kühn, 9:80).

84. Instead of "weakness of the faculty," Galen mentions a "dyscrasy" (δυσκρασία).

85. Galen, *De causis pulsum* 1.6 (ed. Kühn, 9:80).

86. Cf. Galen, *De causis pulsum* 1.6 (ed. Kühn, 9:80): ἡσυχία τηνικαῦτα διακόπτει τὴν διαστολήν (at that time rest interrupts the expansion). Galen actually refers to the characteristics of the pulse called "goat-leap."

87. "When the faculty is in a balanced condition": cf. Galen, *De causis pulsum* 1.6 (ed. Kühn, 9:80): ὅσον μὲν ἐφ' ἑαυτῇ σώζῃ τὸν κατὰ φύσιν τόνον (as long as it keeps its natural force).

88. I.e., arteries.

89. Galen, *De causis pulsum* 1.6 (ed. Kühn, 9:80).

90. I.e, arteries.

91. Cf. Galen, *De causis pulsum* 4 (ed. Kühn, 9:23): ταῖς δ' εἰς ἀραιότητα οἷον διατεθρυμμένος, ἀνωμάλου δυσκρασίας αὐτῶν τῶν ὀργάνων ἔγγονος ὑπάρχων (in the case of others, the pulse that has been broken into pieces so that it has become very rare originates from an unequal bad temperament).

92. Galen, *De causis pulsum* 4 (ed. Kühn, 9:23).

The Fifth Treatise

1. Cf. Galen, *De crisibus* 1.7 (ed. Kühn, 9:579): ἐπειδὴ τοῦ ἰεβώδους γένους εἰσὶ παθήματα.

2. Galen, *De crisibus* 1.7 (ed. Kühn, 9:579–80).

3. Galen, *De differentiis febrium* 1.8 (ed. Kühn, 7:301).

4. Galen, *In Hippocratis Aphorismos commentarius* 8.33 and Galen's commentary on them (ed. Kühn, 18A:133–34).

5. Galen, *In Hippocratis Aphorismos commentarius* 8.34 and Galen's commentary on them (ed. Kühn, 18A:134–35).

6. Galen, *In Hippocratis Aphorismos commentarius* 8.33–34 and Galen's commentary on them (ed. Kühn, 18A:133–35).

7. Galen, *De crisibus* 1.12 (ed. Kühn, 9:598–99).

8. Cf. Galen, *De crisibus* 1.12 (ed. Kühn, 9:604–5): Τὰ μὲν δὴ τοιαῦτα τῶν οὔρων μοχθηρά, τὰ δ' εὔχροά θ' ἅμα καὶ ἤτοι τὰς ὑποστάσεις λευκὰς καὶ λείας καὶ ὁμαλὰς ἢ νεφέλας τινὰς ὁμοίας ἢ ἐναιωρήματα ποιούμενα πάντων ἐστὶν οὔρων τὰ χρηστότατα, μάλιστα μὲν ὧν ἡ ὑπόστασίς ἐστι τοιαύτη, δεύτερα δ' ὧν ἐναιωρήματα, τρίτα δ' ὧν αἱ νεφέλαι. (But urine of a proper colour, and which at the same time has white, smooth, and equable sediments, or certain cloud-like appearances, or substances swimming in the middle of a like kind, is of all others the best. Of these characters, the sediment is of the most importance; next, the substances swimming in it; and third, the cloud-like appearances on its surface"). Cf. Adams, trans., *The Seven Books of Paulus Aegineta* 1.14 (1:225).

9. Meaning crudity. The Greek reads ἀπεψία. Galen, *De crisibus* 1.12 (ed. Kühn, 9:605).

10. Greek: ὀλέθρον. Galen, *De crisibus* 1.12 (ed. Kühn, 9:605).

11. Galen, *De crisibus* 1.12 (ed. Kühn, 9:604–5).

12. Greek ἡμιπέπτος. Galen, *De crisibus* 1.12 (ed. Kühn, 9:606).

13. Galen, *De crisibus* 1.12 (ed. Kühn, 9:605–6).

14. Galen, *De crisibus* 1.12 (ed. Kühn, 9:594–96).

15. "Small amount" *(al-iqlāl)* is a translation of the Greek ἐνδεία. Galen, *De crisibus* 1.12 (ed. Kühn, 9:602).

16. Galen, *De crisibus* 1.12 (ed. Kühn, 9:602).

17. Galen, *In Hippocratis Prognostica commentarius* 2.26 (ed. Kühn, 18B:148–49).

18. "Truly" *(ʿalā al-ṣiḥḥa)* is a translation of the Greek ἀκριβῶς. Galen, *De crisibus* 1.12 (ed. Kühn, 9:596).

19. Galen, *De crisibus* 1.12 (ed. Kühn, 9:595–96).

20. Galen, *De locis affectis* 6.3 (ed. Kühn, 8:394).

21. "Diarrhea" *(ikhtilāf)* is a translation of the Greek διαχωρήματα (excrements). Galen, *In Hipp. Epid. 1 & 2,* 163 lines 1–2.

22. Cf. ibid., 163 lines 1–16; trans. Deller, 530, no. 51.

23. Galen, *De crisibus* 1.12 (ed. Kühn, 9:597).

24. Cf. Galen, *De crisibus* 1.12 (ed. Kühn, 9:604): πελιδνὸν δὲ χρῶμα.

25. Galen, *De crisibus* 1.12 (ed. Kühn, 9:603–4).

26. Galen, *De crisibus* 1.12 (ed. Kühn, 9:604).

27. Cf. Galen, *De totius morbi temporibus* 6 (ed. Kühn, 8:457): καὶ μᾶλλον εἰ καὶ σύμπαν εἴη ζοφῶδες (especially when it is totally dark).

28. "Cereal" *(sawīq):* semolina. "It is wheat, barley and other similar roasted cereals, agitated with butter and then ground"; Maimonides, *Drug Names,* ed. and trans. Rosner, no. 284. The Greek term used is κριμνώδη. Galen, *De totius morbi temporibus* 6 (ed. Kühn, 8:457).

29. "Flakes" *(safā'iḥ):* literally, "leaves" or "flakes." It is a translation of the Greek πεταλώδη. Galen, *De totius morbi temporibus* 6 (ed. Kühn, 8:457).

30. Galen, *De totius morbi temporibus* 6 (ed. Kühn, 8:457).

31. Galen, *De crisibus* 1.12 (ed. Kühn, 9:604–5).

32. "Slow to move": the Greek reads βραδύ. Galen, *De crisibus* 3.11 (ed. Kühn, 9:761).

33. "Most likely" *(al-akhlaq),* which translates the Greek μᾶλλον εἰκὸς. Galen, *De crisibus* 3.11 (ed. Kühn, 9:761).

34. Galen, *De crisibus* 3.11 (ed. Kühn, 9:761).

35. See Dietrich, trans. and ed., *Dioscurides triumphans,* 2:256 (2.92); Maimonides, *Drug Names,* ed. and trans. Rosner, no. 185.

36. Galen, *In Hipp. Epid.* 6, 294 line 20 reads κριμνοειδῆ (like coarse meal).

37. Galen, ibid., 294 lines 20–28; trans. Deller, 538, no. 8.

Bibliographies

Translations and Editions of Works by or Attributed to Moses Maimonides

(arranged alphabetically by translator or editor)

Avishur, Yitzhak, ed. *Shivḥe ha-Rambam: Sippurim ᶜamamiyim be-ᶜArvit Yehudit uve-ᶜIvrit meha Mizraḥ umi-Tsefon ᵓAfriḳah.* Jerusalem: Magnes Press, 1998.

Bar-Sela, Ariel, Hebbel E. Hoff, and Elias Faris, trans. and eds. *Moses Maimonides' Two Treatises on the Regimen of Health:* Fī tadbīr al-ṣiḥḥa *and* Maqāla fī bayān baᶜḍ al-aᶜrāḍ wa-al-jawāb ᶜanhā. Transactions of the American Philosophical Society, New Series, 54.4. Philadelphia: American Philosophical Society, 1964.

Barzel, Uriel S., trans. and ed. *The Art of Cure: Extracts from Galen.* Maimonides' Medical Writings, [5]. Foreword by Fred Rosner; bibliography by Jacob I. Dienstag. Haifa: Maimonides Research Institute, 1992.

Bos, Gerrit, ed. and trans. *Medical Aphorisms,* 5 vols. Forthcoming.

———, ed. and trans. *On Asthma.* Provo, Utah: Brigham Young University Press, 2002.

Deller, K. H. "Die Exzerpte des Moses Maimonides aus den Epidemienkommentaren des Galen." Supplement to Galen, *In Hippocratis Epidemiarum librum VI commentaria I–VIII.* Ed. Ernst Wenkebach and Franz Pfaff. Berlin: Academia Litterarum, 1956.

Ferre, Lola, ed. and trans. *El régimen de salud: Tratado sobre la curación de las hemorroides.* Maimonides obras médicas, 1. Córdoba: Ediciones el Almendro, 1991.

Gorlin, Morris, trans. and ed. *On Sexual Intercourse:* Fī al-jimāᶜ. Medical Historical Studies of Medieval Jewish Medical Works, 1. Brooklyn, N.Y.: Rambash, 1961.

Ḳafaḥ, Yosef, ed. *Igrot: Maḳor ṿe-targum.* 1972; reprint, Jerusalem: Mosad ha-Rav Ḳuḳ, 1987.

Kroner, Hermann, ed. "Der medicinische Schwanengesang des Maimonides: *Fī bajān al-aᶜrāḍ* (Über die Erklärung der Zufälle)." *Janus* 32 (1928): 12–116.

———, ed. and trans. "Die Haemorrhoiden in der Medicin des XII und XIII Jahrhunderts . . . ." *Janus* 16 (1911): 441–56, 645–718.

———, ed. and trans. "Eine medizinische Maimonides-Handschrift aus Granada." *Janus* 21 (1916): 203–47.

———, ed. and trans. "*Fī tadbīr al-ṣiḥḥa:* Gesundheitsanleitung des Maimonides für den Sultan al-Malik al-Afḍal." *Janus* 27 (1923): 101–16, 286–300; 28 (1924): 61–74, 143–52, 199–217, 408–19, 455–72; 29 (1925): 235–58. Reprinted in *Beiträge zur Geschichte der arabisch-islamischen Medizin: Aufsätze,* ed. Fuat Sezgin, in cooperation with M. Amawi, D. Bischoff, and E. Neubauer, 5 (1921–28): 91–202. Frankfurt am Main: Institut für Geschichte der Arabisch-Islamischen Wissenschaften, Johann Wolfgang Goethe-Universität, 1990.

———, ed. and trans. "Shene maʾamare ha-Mishgal: Eḥad ʿal ʿinyane ha-Mishgal ve ʾeḥad ʿal ribbuy ha-Mishgal." In *Ein Beitrag zur Geschichte der Medizin des XII. Jahrhunderts, an der Hand zweier medizinischer Abhandlungen des Maimonides auf Grund von 6 unedierten Handschriften, dargestellt und kritisch beleuchtet.* [Berlin: Itzkowski,] 1906.

Leibowitz, Joshua O., and Shlomo Marcus, eds., with the collaboration of M. Beit-Arié, E. D. Goldschmidt, F. Klein-Franke, E. Lieber, M. Plessner. *Moses Maimonides on the Causes of Symptoms:* Maqāla fi bayān baʿḍ al-aʿrāḍ wa-al-jawāb ʿanhā, Maʾamar ha-Hakraʾah, De Causis Accidentium. Berkeley and Los Angeles: University of California Press, 1974.

Meyerhof, Max, ed. *Sharḥ asmāʾ al-ʿuqqār (L'explication des noms des drogues): Un glossaire de matière médicale composé par Maïmonide.* Cairo: Imprimerie de l'Institut français d'archéologie orientale, 1940. (See also Rosner's translation below.)

Muntner, Süssmann, ed. *Beʾur shemot refuʾiyot.* Jerusalem: Mosad ha-Rav Ḳuḳ, [1969].

———, ed. *Bi-refu'at ha-teḥorim: Ma'amar ʿal ḥizuḳ koʾaḥ ha-gavra.* Ketavim Refu'iyim 4. Jerusalem: Mosad ha-Rav Ḳuḳ, 1965.

———, ed. *Hanhagat ha-beriʾut.* Trans. Mosheh Ibn Tibbon. Jerusalem: Mosad ha-Rav Ḳuḳ, [1957].

———, ed. *Perush le-firḳe Abuḳrat.* Trans. Mosheh Ibn Tibbon. Jerusalem: Mosad ha-Rav Ḳuḳ, [1961].

———, ed. *Pirḳe Mosheh bi-refuʾah.* Trans. Nathan ha-Meʾati. Jerusalem: Mosad ha-Rav Ḳuḳ, [1959].

———, ed. *Regimen Sanitatis, oder Diätetik für die Seele und den Körper.* Deutsche Übersetzung und Einleitung. Basel: Karger, 1966.

———, ed. *Same ha-maṿet veha-refuʾot ke-negdam.* Trans. Mosheh Ibn Tibbon. Jerusalem: Rubin Mass, [1942].

———, ed. and trans. *Treatise on Poisons and Their Antidotes.* The Medical Writings of Moses Maimonides, 2. Philadelphia: Lippincott, 1966.

Pines, Shlomo, trans. *The Guide of the Perplexed.* 2 vols. Chicago: University of Chicago Press, 1963.

Rabbinowicz, I. M., trans. *Traité des poisons.* 1865. Reprint, Paris: Librairie Upschutz, 1935.

Rosner, Fred, ed. and trans. *Maimonides' Commentary on the Aphorisms of Hippocrates.* Maimonides' Medical Writings, 2. Haifa: Maimonides Research Institute, 1987.

———, trans. *The Medical Aphorisms of Moses Maimonides.* Maimonides' Medical Writings, 3. Haifa: Maimonides Research Institute, 1989.

———, ed. and trans. *Moses Maimonides' Glossary of Drug Names.* Maimonides' Medical Writings, 7. Haifa: Maimonides Research Institute, 1995. (See also Meyerhof's translation above.)

———, ed. and trans. *Moses Maimonides' Three Treatises on Health.* Maimonides' Medical Writings, 4. Haifa: Maimonides Research Institute, 1990.

———, ed. and trans. *Moses Maimonides' Treatise on Asthma.* Maimonides' Medical Writings, 6. Haifa: Maimonides Research Institute, 1994.

———, ed. and trans. *Treatises on Poisons, Hemorrhoids, Cohabitation.* 2nd ed. Maimonides' Medical Writings, 1. Haifa: Maimonides Research Institute, 1988.

Rosner, Fred, and Süssman Muntner, ed. and trans. *The Medical Aphorisms of Moses Maimonides.* 2 pts. in 1 vol. Studies in Judaica, 3. New York: Yeshiva University Press, Department of Special Publications, 1970–71.

———, ed. and trans. *Treatise on Hemorrhoids, Medical Answers (Responsa).* The Medical Writings of Moses Maimonides, 3. Philadelphia: Lippincott, 1969.

Schliwski, C. *Commentary on the Aphorisms of Hippocrates.* Edition and German translation forthcoming.

Shailat, Isaac, ed. *Igrot ha-Rambam.* 2 vols. Jerusalem: Hotsa$^{\circ}$at Ma^{c}aliyot le-yad Yeshivat "Birkat Mosheh" Ma^{c}aleh Adumim, 1987–88.

Steinschneider, Moritz, trans. "Gifte und ihre Heilung: Eine Abhandlung des Moses Maimonides, auf Befehl des Aegyptischen Wezirs (1198) verfasst . . . ." *Virchows Archiv* 57 (1873): 62–120.

Stern, S. M., ed. and trans. "Maimonides' Treatise to a Prince, Containing Advice on Sexual Matters." In *Maimonidis Commentarius in Mischnam . . . ,* ed. S. M. Stern, 17–21. Corpus codicum Hebraicorum Medii Aevi, 1.3. Copenhagen: Ejnar Munksgaard, 1966.

General Bibliography

Ackermann, Hermann. "Moses Maimonides (1135–1204): Ärztliche Tätigkeit und medizinische Schriften." *Sudhoffs Archiv* 70, no. 1 (1986): 44–63.

Anastassiou, Anargyros, and Dieter Irmer, eds. *Testimonien zum Corpus Hippocraticum.* Part 2, Galen. Vol. 1: *Hippokrateszitate in den Kommentaren und im Glossar.* Göttingen, Ger.: Vandenhoeck and Ruprecht, 1997.

Aristotle. *Aristotle's* De anima *Translated into Hebrew by Zeraḥyah ben Isaac ben She$^{\circ}$altiel Ḥen: A Critical Edition with an Introducation and Index.* Ed. Gerrit Bos. Leiden: Brill, 1994.

———. *On the Soul, Parva Naturalia, On Breath.* Trans. Walter S. Hett. Loeb Classical Library. 1936. Reprint, Cambridge, Mass.: Harvard University Press, 1986.

———. *Parts of Animals.* Trans. Arthur L. Peck. *Movement of Animals, Progression of Animals.* Trans. Edward S. Forster. Loeb Classical Library. 1937. Reprint, Cambridge, Mass.: Harvard University Press, 1983.

Averroës. "Averroes 'contra Galenum': Das Kapitel von der Atmung im Colliget des Averroes als ein Zeugnis mittelalterlich-islamischer Kritik an Galen." Ed. and trans. J. Christoph Bürgel. *Nachrichten von der Akademie der Wissenschaften in Göttingen: Philologisch-historische Klasse* 9 (1967): 263–340.

———. *Epitome of Parva Naturalia.* Ed. and trans. Harry Blumberg. Cambridge, Mass.: Mediaeval Academy of America, 1961.

Barkaï, Ron. *Les infortunes de Dinah: Le livre de la génération: La gynécologie juive au Moyen-Age.* Paris: Cerf, 1991.

Baron, Salo Wittmeyer. *High Middle Ages, 500–1200: Philosophy and Science.* Vol. 8 of *A Social and Religious History of the Jews.* 2nd ed., rev. and enl. New York: Columbia University Press, 1952–92.

Beit-Arié, Malachi, comp., and R. A. May, ed. *Catalogue of the Hebrew Manuscripts in the Bodleian Library: Supplement of Addenda and Corrigenda to Vol. 1 (A. Neubauer's Catalogue).* Oxford, Eng.: Clarendon, 1994. (See also Neubauer's catalogue below.)

Ben-Sasson, Menahem. "Maimonides in Egypt: The First Stage." *Maimonidean Studies* 2 (1991): 3–30.

Bergsträsser, Gotthelf. *Neue Materialien zu Ḥunayn ibn Isḥāq's Galen-Bibiographie.* Abhandlungen für die Kunde des Morgenländes 19.2. Leipzig: Deutsche Morgenländische Gesellschaft, 1932.

Blau, Joshua. *The Emergence and Background of Judaeo-Arabic: A Study of the Origins of Middle Arabic.* Scripta Judaica, 5. London: Oxford University Press, 1965.

Bos, Gerrit. *Aristotle's* De anima. *Translated into Hebrew by Zeraḥyah ben Isaac ben She'altiel Ḥen; A Critical Edition with an Introduction and Index.* Leiden: E.J. Brill, 1994.

———. "Ibn al-Jazzār on Sexuality and Sexual Dysfunction and the Mystery of ʿUbaid ibn ʿAlī Ibn Jurāja ibn Ḥillauf Solved." *Jerusalem Studies in Arabic and Islam* 19 (1995): 250–66.

———. "Maimonides' Medical Aphorisms: Towards a Critical Edition and Revised English Translation." *Ḳorot* 12 (1996–97): 35–79.

———. "The Reception of Galen in Maimonides' Medical Aphorisms." In *The Unknown Galen,* ed. Vivian Nutton, 139–52. London: Institute of Classical Studies, University of London, 2002.

———. "A Recovered Fragment on the Signs of Death from Abū Yūsuf al-Kindī's 'Medical Summaries.'" *Zeitschrift für Geschichte der arabisch-islamischen Wissenschaften* 6 (1990): 189–94.

———. "R. Moshe Narboni, Philosopher and Physician: A Critical Analysis of Sefer Oraḥ Ḥayyim." *Medieval Encounters* 1 (1995): 219–51.

Brain, Peter. *Galen on bloodletting: A Study of the Origins, Development and Validity of His Opinions, with a Translation of the Three Works.* Cambridge, Eng.: Cambridge University Press, 1986.

Cano Ledesma, Aurora. *Indización de los manuscritos árabes de El Escorial.* Madrid: Ediciones Escurialenses, Real Biblioteca de El Escorial, 1996.

Cohen, Mark R. "Maimonides' Egypt." In *Moses Maimonides and His Time,* ed. Eric L. Ormsby, 21–34. Studies in Philosophy and the History of Philosophy, 19. Washington, D.C.: The Catholic University of America Press, 1989.

Conrad, Lawrence I. Review of "Medical and Paramedical Manuscripts in the Cambridge Genizah Collections," by Haskell D. Isaacs. *Bulletin of the School of Oriental and African Studies* 59 (1996): 136–37.

Davidson, Herbert. "Maimonides' Putative Position as Official Head of the Egyptian Jewish Community." In *Ḥazon Naḥum, Jubilee Volume,* ed. N. Lamm, 115–28. New York: Yeshiva University, 1998.

De Chauliac, Guy (Guigonis de Caulhiaco). *Inventarium sive chirurgia magna.* 2 vols. Ed. Michael R. McVaugh with commentary by Michael R. McVaugh and Margaret S. Ogden. Leiden: Brill, 1997.

Derenbourg, Hartwig, comp., and H. P. J. Renaud, ed. *Médecine et histoire naturelle.* Vol. 2, fasc. 2 of *Les manuscrits arabes de l'Escurial.* Publications de l'Ecole nationale des langues orientales vivantes. Paris: LeRoux, 1939.

Dienstag, Jacob I. "Bibliography of the Medical Aphorisms of Maimonides." Appendix to Maimonides, *The Medical Aphorisms of Moses Maimonides.* Trans. Fred Rosner. Maimoides' Medical Writings, vol. 1. Haifa: Maimonides Research Institute, 1989.

———. "Translators and Editors of Maimonides' Medical Works." In *Memorial Volume in Honor of Professor Süssmann Muntner,* ed. Joshua O. Leibowitz, 95–135. Jerusalem: Israel Institute for the History of Medicine, 1983.

Dietrich, Albert, trans. and ed. *Dioscurides triumphans: Ein anonymer arabischer Kommentar (Ende 12. Jahrh. n. Chr.) zur* Materia medica. 2 vols. Abhandlungen der Akademie der Wissenschaften in Göttingen, Philologisch-Historische Klasse, Dritte Folge, 172. Göttingen: Vandenhoeck and Ruprecht, 1988.

Dols, Michael W. *Majnūn: The Madman in Medieval Islamic Society.* Ed. Diana E. Immisch. Oxford: Clarendon, 1992.

Dozy, R. P. A. *Supplément aux dictionnaires arabes.* 2nd ed. 2 vols. Leiden: Brill, 1927.

Efros, Israel. *Philosophical Terms in the Moreh Nebukim.* Columbia University Oriental Studies, 22. New York: AMS, 1924.

Encyclopaedia Judaica. 16 vols. Jerusalem: Keter, 1971.

Encyclopaedia of Islam. New ed. 10ff. vols. Leiden: Brill, 1960–.

Endress, Gerhard, and Dimitri Gutas, eds. *A Greek and Arabic Lexicon (GALex): Materials for a Dictionary of the Mediaeval Translations from Greek into Arabic.* Fasc. 1ff. Leiden: Brill, 1992–.

Friedenwald, Harry. *The Jews and Medicine: Essays.* 2 vols. 1944. Reprint, New York: Johns Hopkins University Press, 1967.

Galen. *Claudii Galeni opera omnia.* Ed. C. G. Kühn. 20 vols. 1821–33. Reprint, Hildesheim, Ger.: Olms, 1964–67.

———. *De alimentorum facultatibus.* Ed. G. Helmreich. Corpus Medicorum Graecorum, 5.4.2. Leipzig: Teubner, 1923.

———. *De atra bile.* Ed. Wilko de Boer. Corpus Medicorum Graecorum, 5.4.1.1. Leipzig: Teubner, 1937.

———. *De bonis malisque sucis.* Ed. G. Helmreich. Corpus Medicorum Graecorum, 5.4.2. Leipzig: Teubner, 1923.

———. *De instrumento odoratus.* Ed. and trans. Jutta Kollesch. Galen über das Riechorgan. Corpus Medicorum Graecorum, 5. Berlin: Akademie, 1964.

———. *De Marcore.* See "Galen on Marasmus."

———. *De naturalibus facultatibus.* In *Claudii Galeni Pergameni Scripta Minora.* Ed. J. Marquardt, I. Mueller, and G. Helmreich. Leipzig: Teubner, 1884.
———. *De sanitate tuenda.* Ed. K. Koch. Corpus Medicorum Graecorum, 5.4.2. Leipzig: Teubner, 1923. (See also Green's translation below.)
———. *De somno et vigilia.* See Galen. "Die ps.-galenische Schrift 'Über Schlaf und Wachsein.' "
———. *De usu partium.* Ed. Georg Helmreich. 2 vols. Bibliotheca Scriptorum Graecorum et Romanorum Teubneriana. Leipzig: Teubner, 1907–9. (See also May's translation below.)
———. "Die ps.-galenische Schrift 'Über Schlaf und Wachsein' sum ersten Male herausgegeben, übersetzt und erläutert." Ed and trans. R. Nabielek. Ph.D. diss., Humboldt-Universität zu Berlin, 1977.
———. *Exhortation à l'etude de la medicine: Art médical.* Ed. and trans. Véronique Boudon. Paris: Les Belles Lettres, 2000.
———. "Galen on Nerves, Veins, and Arteries." Trans. Emilie Savage-Smith. Ph.D. diss., University of Wisconsin, 1969.
———. *Galen on the Affected Parts.* Trans. Rudolph E. Siegel. New York: Karger, 1976.
———. *Galen's Commentary on the Hippocratic Treatise* Airs, Waters, Places: *In the Hebrew Translation of Solomon ha-Me'ati.* Ed. and trans. Abraham Wasserstein. Proceedings of the Israel Academy of Sciences and Humanities 6, no. 3 (1983).
———. "Galen on Marasmus." Trans. Theoharis C. Theoharides. *Journal of the History of Medicine* 26, no. 4 (1971): 369–90.
———. *In Hippocratis De natura hominis commentaria tria.* Ed. I. Mewaldt. Corpus Medicorum Graecorum, 5.9.1. Leipzig: Teubner, 1914.
———. *Galeni in Hippocratis Epidemiarum libros I et II.* Ed. Ernst Wenkebach and Franz Pfaff. Corpus medicorum Graecorum, V.10.1. Leipzig: Teubner, 1934.
———. *Galeni in Hippocratis Epidemiarum librum III commentaria III.* Ed. Ernst Wenkebach. Corpus medicorum Graecorum, V.10.2.1. Leipzig: Teubner, 1936.
———. *Galeni in Hippocratis Epidemiarum librum VI commentaria I–VIII.* Ed. Ernst Wenkebach and Franz Pfaff. Corpus medicorum Graecorum, V.10.2.2. Berlin: Academiae Litterarum, 1956.
———. "On Movement of Muscles." Trans. Charles Mayo Goss. *American Journal of Anatomy* 123, no. 1 (1968): 1–25.
———. *On Respiration and the Arteries.* Trans. David J. Furley and J. S. Wilkie. Princeton, N.J.: Princeton University Press, 1984.
———. *On Semen.* Ed. and trans. Phillip De Lacy. Corpus Medicorum Graecorum, 5.3.1. Berlin: Akademie, 1992.
———. *On the Doctrines of Hippocrates and Plato.* Ed. and trans. Phillip de Lacy. 3 vols. Corpus Medicorum Graecorum, 5.4.1.2. Berlin: Akademie-Verlag, 1978–84.
———. *On the Natural Faculties.* Trans. Arthur John Brock. Loeb Classical Library. 1916. Reprint, Cambridge, Mass.: Harvard University Press, 1979.

———. *On the Usefulness of the Parts of the Body.* Trans. Margaret Tallmadge May. 2 vols. Ithaca, N.Y.: Cornell University Press, 1968. (See also Helmreich's edition above.)

———. *A Translation of Galen's* Hygiene. Trans. Robert Montraville Green. Introduction by Henry E. Sigerist. Springfield, Ill.: Thomas, 1951. (See also Koch's edition above.)

García-Ballester, Luis. "The New Galen: A Challenge to Latin Galenism in Thirteenth-Century Montpellier." In *Text and Tradition: Studies in Ancient Medicine and its Transmission, Presented to Jutta Kollesch.* Ed. Klaus-Dietrich Fischer, Diethard Nickel, and Paul Potter, 55–83. Studies in Ancient Medicine 18. Leiden: Brill, 1988.

Goitein, Shelomoh-D. "Ḥayyē ha-Rambam le-ᵓOr Gilluyim ḥadashim min ha-genizah ha-ḳahirit." *Peraḳim* 4 (1966): 29–42.

———. "Moses Maimonides, Man of Action: A Revision of the Master's Biography in Light of the Geniza Documents." In *Hommage à Georges Vajda: Études d'histoire et de pensée juives,* ed. Gérard Nahon and Charles Touati, 155–67. Louvain, Belg.: Éditions Peeters, 1980.

Graetz, Heinrich. *Geschichte der Juden.* 11 vols. Leipzig: Leiner, 1890–1909.

Gross, Henri. *Gallia Judaica: Dictionnaire géographique de la France d'après les sources rabbiniques. Traduit sur le manuscript de l'auteur par Moïse Bloch.* Paris: Librairie Léopold Cerf, 1897.

Hippocrates. *Aphorisms.* Trans. W. H. S. Jones. Loeb Classical Library. 1931. Reprint, Cambridge, Mass.: Harvard University Press, 1979.

———. *Oeuvres complètes d'Hippocrate.* Trans. É. Littré. 10 vols. 1839–61. Reprint, Amsterdam: Hakkert, 1973–89.

Ibn Abī Uṣaybiᶜa. *ᶜUyūn al-anbāᵓ fī ṭabaqāt al-aṭibbāᵓ.* Beirut: Dār Maktabat al-Ḥayāt, n.d.

Ibn al-Jazzār. *Ibn al-Jazzār on Sexual Diseases and Their Treatment: A Critical Edition of* Zād al-musāfir wa-qūt al-ḥāḍir. Trans. and ed. Gerrit Bos. London: Kegan Paul, 1997.

Ibn Falaquera, Shem Tov ben Joseph. *Moreh ha-moreh.* Ed. Yair Shiffman. Jerusalem: World Union of Jewish Studies, 2001.

Ibn Ishaq, Hunayn. *Ḥunain ibn Isḥāq über die syrischen und arabischen Galen-Übersetzungen.* Trans. and ed. G. Bergstrasser. Leipzig: Brockhaus, 1925.

Ibn Māsawayh, Yūḥannā. *Le livre des axiomes médicaux (Aphorismi).* Ed. and trans. Danielle Jacquart and Gérard Troupeau. Hautes études orientales, 14. Geneva: Droz, 1980.

Ibn Sahl, Sābūr. *Dispensatorium parvum (Al-aqrābādhīn al-ṣaghīr).* Ed. Oliver Kahl. Islamic Philosophy, Theology, and Science: Texts and Studies, 16. Leiden: Brill, 1994.

Ibn Wāfid of Toledo. *"El Libro de la Almohada" de Ibn Wafid de Toledo.* Trans. Camilo Alvarez de Morales y Ruiz-Matas. Toledo: Instituto Provincial de Investigaciones y Estudios Toledanos, 1980.

Kahle, Paul. "Mosis Maimonidis Aphorismum Praefatio et Excerpta." In *Galeni in Platonis Timaeum commentarii fragmenta,* ed. Heinrich Otto Schröder. Corpus Medicorum Graecorum, Supp. 1. Berlin: Teubner, 1934.

Kaufmann, David. "Le neveu de Maïmonide." *Revue des études juives* 7 (1883): 152–53.

Kraemer, Joel L. "The Life of Moses ben Maimon." In *Judaism in Practice: From the Middle Ages through the Early Modern Period,* ed. Lawrence Fine, 413–28. Princeton, N.J.: Princeton University Press, 2001.

———. "Six Unpublished Maimonides Letters from the Cairo Genizah." In *Maimonidean Studies,* vol. 2, ed. A. Hyman, 61–94. New York: Yeshiva University Press, 1991.

Kroner, Hermann. *Zur Terminologie der arabischen Medizin und zu ihrem zeitgenössischen hebräischen Ausdrucke . . .* Berlin: Itzkowski, 1921.

Lane, Edward William. *Arabic-English Lexicon.* London: Williams and Norgate, 1863–79.

Langermann, Y. Tzvi. "Arabic Writings in Hebrew Manuscripts: A Preliminary Listing." *Arabic Sciences and Philosophy* 6, no. 1 (March 1996): 137–60.

———. "Maimonides on the Synochous Fever." *Israel Oriental Studies* 13 (1993): 175–98.

Larrain, Carlos J. "Galen, De motibus dubiis: Die lateinische Übersetzung des Niccolò da Reggio." *Traditio* 49 (1994): 171–233.

Leibowitz, Joshua O. "The Latin Translations of Maimonides' Aphorisms." *Ḳorot* 6 (1970): xciii–xciv, 273–81.

———. "Maimonides: Der Mann und sein Werk: Formen der Weisheit." *Ariel,* no. 40 (1976): 73–89.

———. "Maimonides' Aphorisms." *Ḳorot* 1 (1955): 213–19 Hebrew; i–iii English.

———. "Verschiedene Arten der Weisheit II: Maimonides in der Geschichte der Medizin." *Ariel,* no. 41 (1976): 37–52.

Levinger, Jacob. "Was Maimonides 'Rais al-Yahud' in Egypt?" In *Studies in Maimonides,* ed. Isadore Twersky, 83–93. Harvard Judaic Texts and Studies, 7. Cambridge, Mass.: Harvard University Center for Jewish Studies, 1990.

Lewis, Bernard."Maimonides, Lionheart and Saladin." In *ʾEreṣ-Yiśrāʾēl: Archaeological, Historical, and Geographical Studies,* vol. 7, ed. M. Avi-Yonah, H. Z. Hirschberg, B. Mazar, and Y. Yadin, 70–75. Jerusalem: Israel Exploration Society, 1964.

Lieber, Elinor. "Maimonides, the Medical Humanist." *Maimonidean Studies* 4 (2000): 39–60.

———. "The Medical Works of Maimonides: A Reappraisal." In *Moses Maimonides: Physician, Scientist, and Philosopher,* ed. Fred Rosner and Samuel S. Kottek, 13–24. North Vale, N. J.: Aronson, 1993.

Meyerhof, Max. "The Medical Work of Maimonides." In *Essays on Maimonides: An Octocentennial Volume,* ed. Salo Wittmayer Baron, 265–99. New York: Columbia University Press, 1941.

———. "Über echte und unechte Schriften Galens, nach arabischen Quellen." *Sitzungsberichte der Preussischen Akademie der Wissenschaften: Philosophisch-historische Klasse* 28 (1928): 533–48.

Neubauer, Adolf. *Catalogue of the Hebrew Manuscripts in the Bodleian Library and in the College Libararies of Oxford.* 1886. Reprint, Oxford: Clarendon, 1994. (See also Beit-Arié's supplement above.)

Niebyl, P. H. "Old Age, Fever, and the Lamp Metaphor." *Journal of the History of Medicine* 26 (1971): 351–68.

Paulus Aegineta. *The Seven Books of Paulus Aegineta.* Trans. Francis Adams. 3 vols. London: Sydenham Society, 1844–47.

Pertsch, Wilhelm. *Die orientalischen Handschriften der Herzoglichen Bibliothek zu Gotha.* Part 3, *Die arabischen Handschriften.* Vols. 1–5. Gotha: Perthes, 1877–92.

Ravitzky, Aviezer. "Mishnato shel R. Zeraḥyah ben Isaac ben She'altiel Ḥen." Ph.D. diss., Hebrew University, 1977.

al-Rāzī, Abū Bakr. *Kitāb al-murshid aw al-fuṣūl.* Ed. A. Z. Iskandar. In *Revue de l'Institut des manuscrits arabes* 7, no. 1 (May 1961).

Renan, E. *Les écrivains juifs français du XIVe siècle.* 1893. Reprint, Farnborough, Eng.: Gregg, 1969.

Richler, Benjamin. "Another Letter from Hillel ben Samuel to Isaac the Physician?" *Kiryat Sefer* 62, nos. 1–2 (1988–89): 450–52.

———, ed. *Hebrew Manuscripts in the Bibliotheca Palatina in Parma.* With palaeographical and codicological descriptions by M. Beit-Arié. Jerusalem: Hebrew University of Jerusalem/Jewish National and University Library, 2001.

———. "Manuscripts of Moses ben Maimon's Pirke Moshe in Hebrew translation," *Ḳorot* 9, nos. 3–4 (1986): 345–56.

Richter-Bernburg, Lutz, trans. "Eine arabische Version der pseudogalenischen Schrift *De Theriaca ad Pisonem.*" Ph.D. diss., University of Göttingen, 1969.

Rosner, Fred. "Medical Writings of Moses Maimonides." *New York State Journal of Medicine* 73 (1 September 1973): 2185–90.

———. *Sex Ethics in the Writings of Moses Maimonides.* New York: Bloch, 1974.

———. "The Medical Aphorisms of Maimonides." In *Memorial Volume in Honor of Professor Süssmann Muntner,* ed. Joshua O. Leibowitz, 6–30. Jerusalem: Israel Institute for the History of Medicine, 1983.

Schacht, J., and M. Meyerhof. "Maimonides against Galen, on Philosophy and Cosmogony." *Bulletin of the Faculty of Arts of the University of Egypt* 5, no. 1 (1937): 53–88 (Arabic section).

Sezgin, Fuat. *Medizin-Pharmazie-Zoologie-Tierheilkunde bis ca. 430 H.* Vol. 3 of *Geschichte des arabischen Schrifttums.* Leiden: Brill, 1970.

Shatzmiller, Joseph. *Jews, Medicine, and Medieval Society.* Berkeley: University of California Press, 1994.

Sirat, C. "Une liste de manuscrits du Dalālat al-ḥayryn." *Maimonidean Studies* 4 (2000): 109–33.

Steinschneider, Moritz. *Catalog der hebräischen Handschriften in der Stadtbibliothek zu Hamburg und der sich anschliessenden in anderen Sprachen.* 1878. Reprint, with a foreword by Hellmut Braun, Hildesheim: Olms, 1969.

———. "Die griechischen Ärzte in arabischen Übersetzungen." *Virchows Archiv* 124 (1891): 115–36, 268–96, 455–87.

———. *Die hebräischen Handschriften der K. Hof- und Staatsbibliothek in München.* 2nd ed., rev. and enl. Munich: Palm'sche Hofbuchhandlung, 1895.

———. *Die hebräischen Übersetzungen des Mittelalters und die Juden als Dolmetscher.* 1893. Reprint, Graz, Austria: Akademische Druck- und Verlagsanstalt, 1956.

———. "Eine altfranzösische Compilation eines Juden über die Fieber." *Virchows Archiv* 136 (1894): 399–402.
———. *Verzeichniss der hebräischen Handschriften in Berlin.* 2 vols. 1878–97. Reprint, in 1 vol., Hildesheim, Ger.: Olms, 1980.
Strohmaier, G. "Der syrische und arabische Galen." *Aufstieg und Niedergang der Römischen Welt* 37.2 1987. Part 2, *Principat,* 37.2. Berlin: de Gruyter, 1994.
Ullmann, Manfred. *Die Medizin im Islam.* Handbuch der Orientalistik 1, Ergänzungsband 6.1. Leiden: Brill, 1970.
———. "Zwei spätantike Kommentare zu der hippokratischen Schrift 'De morbis muliebribus.'" *Medizinhistorisches Journal* 12 (1977): 245–62.
Urbach, Ephraim E. *The Sages: Their Concepts and Beliefs.* Trans. Israel Abrahams. 2nd ed. 2 vols. Jerusalem: Magnes, 1979.
Vajda, Georges. *Index général des manuscrits arabes musulmans de la Bibliothèque nationale de Paris.* Publication de l'Institut de recherche et d'histoire des textes, 4. Paris: Éditions du Centre national de la recherche scientifique, 1953.
Veltri, G. *Magie und Halakha: Ansätze zu einem empirischen Wissenschaftsbegriff im spätantiken und frühmittelalterlichen Judentum.* Tübingen, Ger.: Mohr, 1997.
Vogelstein, Hermann, and Paul Rieger. *Geschichte der Juden in Rom.* 2 vols. Berlin: Mayer und Müller, 1895–96.
Voorhoeve, P., comp. *Handlist of Arabic Manuscripts in the Library of the University of Leiden and Other Collections in the Netherlands.* 2nd ed., enl. The Hague: Leiden University Press, 1980.
Wiedemann, Eilhard. *Aufsätze zur arabischen Wissenschafts-geschichte.* 2 vols. Hildesheim, Ger.: Olms, 1970.
Wörterbuch der klassischen arabischen Sprache. Ed. Deutsche Morgenländische Gessellschaft et al. Wiesbaden: Harrassowitz, 1957–.
Zotenberg, H., ed. *Catalogues des manuscrits hébreux et samaritains de la Bibliothèque impériale.* Paris: Imprimerie impériale, 1866.
Zwiep, Irene E. *Mother of Reason and Revelation: A Short History of Medieval Jewish Linguistic Thought.* Amsterdam: Gieben, 1997.

Index of Galenic Passages Cited

Note that some of the titles below are referred to differently by Maimonides in his aphorisms. Such titles are correlated in the notes and in the Index of Galenic Titles. Parentheses contain references to the cited passages as found in modern editions of Galen's works. If the published title (as listed in the bibliography under Galen*) is not identical with the title given below, it will also be listed in the table of abbreviations (p. xii).*

TREATISE — APHORISM

Ad Glauconem de methodo medendi (ed. Kühn)
2.9 (11:116) 3.61

De alimentorum facultatibus (ed. Helmreich)
1.1 (207 lines 9–14) 2.11
1.2 (221 lines 9–16) 2.17
3.1 (333 line 5) 2.16
3.15 (348 lines 12–15) 1.16
3.16 (351 line 28; 352 line 4) 1.17

De anatomia vivorum
2 . . . . 1.49

De arte parva
16 (ed. Kühn, 1:347; ed. Boudon, 323–24) 3.20

De atra bile
2 (ed. Kühn, 5:109–10; ed. de Boer, 73–74) 2.3
3 (ed. Kühn, 5:110–11; ed. de Boer, 74–75) 2.14
7 (ed. Kühn, 5:136; ed. de Boer, 136) 3.50

De causis morborum (ed. Kühn)
6 (7:21–22) 2.12
6 (7:26) 2.22

TREATISE	APHORISM
3.9 (9:742)	3.101
3.9 (9:745)	3.103
3.11 (9:759–68)	3.102
3.11 (9:761)	5.18
3.11 (9:763–64)	4.29
De curandi ratione per venae sectionem (ed. Kühn)	
5 (11:262)	3.46
7 (11:273)	3.8
8 (11:275)	3.56
9 (11:279)	3.11
13 (11:291)	4.4
De differentia pulsuum (ed. Kühn)	
1.6 (8:512)	4.2
1.26 (8:553)	4.33
7.3 (8:907)	4.3
De differentia febrium (ed. Kühn)	
1.6 (7:290–91)	3.68
1.7 (7:299–300)	3.59
1.8 (7:301)	5.2
1.9 (7:306–7)	4.19
1.9 (7:311–12)	4.35
2.6 (7:348–49)	2.6
De dignoscendis pulsibus (ed. Kühn)	
1.5, 9 (8:795, 816)	4.14
1.5 (8:795–96)	4.13
1.11 (8:819–20, 21)	4.36
3.2 (8:888–99)	4.44
4.1 (8:922)	4.12
De inaequali intemperie (ed. Kühn)	
1 (7:733)	3.27
3 (7:736–37)	3.64
De instrumento odoratus	
De instrumento odoratus[1]	1.41
De locis affectis (ed. Kühn)	
3.9 (8:175–76)	2.13
3.9 (8:176–77)	2.15
4.3 (8:229)	1.45
4.6 (8:241)	1.46
4.9 (8:266–67)	1.47

1. Maimonides' quotation does not appear in this text which has not been preserved in the Arabic tradition.

Index of Galenic Titles

Greek, Latin, and transliterated Arabic titles are given according to Gerhard Fichtner, ed., Corpus Galenicum: Verzeichnis der galenischen und pseudogalenischen Schriften *(Tübingen: Institut für Geschichte der Medizin, 1989). Missing titles are indicated by [. . .] following Manfred Ullmann,* Die Medizin im Islam *(Leiden/Cologne: Brill, 1970).*

GREEK TITLE	LATIN TITLE	ARABIC TITLE	MAIMONIDES
[Εἰς τὸ Ἱπποκράτους περὶ ἀέρων ὑδάτων τόπων ὑπομνήματα]	*In Hippocratis De aeris aquis locis commentarius*	Tafsīr K. Buqrāṭ fī l-Ahwiya wa-l-buldān	شرح الأهوية
Εἰς τὸ Ἱπποκράτους περὶ τροφῆς ὑπομνήματα δ′	*In Hippocratis De alimento commentarius*	Tafsīr K. al-ġiḏā᾽	شرح الغذاء
Θεραπευτικῆς μεθόδου βιβλία ιδ′	*De methodo medendi*	K. ḥīlat al-bur᾽ = K. aṣ-ṣināʿa al-kabīra	الحيلة
Ἱπποκράτους ἀφορισμοὶ καὶ Γαληνοῦ εἰς αὐτοὺς ὑπομνήματα	*In Hippocratis Aphorismos commentarius*	Tafsīr K. Fuṣūl Buqrāṭ	شرح الفصول

GREEK TITLE	LATIN TITLE	ARABIC TITLE	MAIMONIDES
Ἱπποκράτους ἐπιδημιῶν α′ καὶ Γαληνοῦ εἰς αὐτὸ ὑπομνήματα γ′, Ἱπποκράτους ἐπιδημιῶν β′ καὶ Γαληνοῦ εἰς αὐτὸ ὑπομνήματα ε′, Ἱπποκράτους ἐπιδημιῶν γ′ καὶ Γαληνοῦ εἰς αὐτὸ ὑπομνήματα ε′, Ἱπποκράτους ἐπιδημιῶν ζ′ καὶ Γαληνοῦ εἰς αὐτὸ ὑπομνήματα, Ἱπποκράτους ἐπιδημιῶν στ′ καὶ Γαληνοῦ εἰς αὐτὸ ὑπομνήματα	*In Hippocratis Epidemiarum libros commentarius*	Tafsīr K. Abīḏīmiyā	شرح ابيديميا
Ἱπποκράτους περὶ φύσιος ἀνθρώπου βιβλίον πρῶτον καὶ Γαληνοῦ εἰς αὐτὸ ὑπομνήμα	*In Hippocratis De natura hominis commentarius*	Tafsīr K. Tadbīr al-amrāḍ al-ḥādda (?) [Tafsīr Jālīnūs li-K. ṭabīʿat al-insān]	شرح طبيعة الإنسان
Ἱπποκράτους προγνοστικὸν καί Γαληνοῦ εἰς αὐτὸ ὑπομνήματα γ′	*In Hippocratis Prognostica commentarius*	Tafsīr Buqrāṭ fī Taqdimat al-maʿrifa	شرح تقدمة المعرفة
Περὶ ἀνωμάλου δυσκρασίας βιβλίον	*De inaequali intemperie liber*	Maq. fī Sūʾ al-mizāj al-muḫtalif	في سوء المزاج المختلف
Περὶ ἀρίστης κατασκευῆς τοῦ σώματος ἡμῶν	*De optima corporis nostri constitutione*	Maq. fī Afḍal haiʾāt al-badan	في أفضل الهيئات
Περὶ διαφορᾶς νοσημάτων βιβλίον, Περὶ τῶν ἐν τοῖς νοσήμασιν αἰτίων βιβλίον, Περὶ συμπτωμάτων διαφορᾶς βιβλίον, Περὶ αἰτίων συμπτωμάτων βιβλία γ′	*De morborum causis et symptomatibus*	K. al-ʿIlal wa-l-aʿrāḍ	العلل والأعراض

GREEK TITLE	LATIN TITLE	ARABIC TITLE	MAIMONIDES
Περὶ δυνάμεων φυσικῶν βιβλία γ′	*De naturalibus facultatibus*	K. al-Quwā ṭ-ṭabīᶜīya	القوى
Περὶ εὐχυμίας καὶ κακοχυμίας τροφῶν	*De probis malisque alimentorum sucis*	K. fī l-Kaimūs al-jayyid wa-r-radīʾ = K. al-Kaimūsain	الكيموس الجيّد والرديء
Περὶ κράσεως καὶ δυνάμεως τῶν ἁπλῶν φαρμάκων βιβλία	*De medicamentis (= De simplicium medicamentorum temperamentis ac facultatibus)*	K. al-Adwiya al-mufrada = K. al-Adwiya al-basīṭa = K. al-Basāʾiṭ	الأدوية
Περὶ κρίσεων βιβλία γ′	*De crisibus*	K. al-Buḥrān = K. al-Buḥrānāt	البحران
Περὶ μαρασμοῦ βιβλίον	*De marcore*	K. aḏ-ḏubūl = Maq. fī s-Sill	في الذبول
Περὶ μελαίνης χολῆς	*De atra bile*	Maq. fī l-Mirra as-saudāʾ	في المرّة السوداء
Περὶ μυῶν κινήσεως βιβλία β′	*De motu musculorum*	K. ḥarakat al-ᶜaḍal	حركات العضل
Περὶ ὀσφρήσεως ὀργάνου	*De instrumento odoratus*	K. fī ālat ash-shamm	في آلة الشمّ
Περὶ πλήθους βιβλίον	*De plenitudine liber*	Maq. fī l-Imtilāʾ	في الكثرة
Περὶ προνοίας	*De providentia creatoris*	Maq. fī ᶜInāyat al-ḫāliq	في عناية الخالق
Περὶ πυρετῶν	*De febribus*	[K. al-ḥummayāt = K. Aṣnāf al-ḥummayāt]	الحمّيات
Περὶ σπέρματος βιβλία β′	*De semine*	K. al-Manī	في المني
Περὶ συνθέσεως φαρμάκων τῶν κατὰ γένη βιβλία	*Qatājānas (De compositione medicamentorum per genera)*	K. fī Tarkīb al-adwiya ᶜalā l-jumal wa-l-ajnās = K. Qāṭājānas	قطاجانس

GREEK TITLE	LATIN TITLE	ARABIC TITLE	MAIMONIDES
Περὶ συνθέσεως φαρμάκων τῶν κατὰ τόπους βιβλία	*Mayāmir (= De compositione medicamentorum secundum locos)*	K. fī Tarkīb al-adwiya bi-ḥasab al-mawāḍi[c] = K. al-mayāmir	الميامر
Περὶ σφυγμῶν	*De pulsu*	. . .	النبض
Περὶ τῆς ἐπὶ τῶν ζώντων ἀνατομῆς	*De anatomia vivorum*	K. Tashrīḥ al-ḥayawān = K. Tashrīḥ al-aḥyā[ɔ]	تشريح الأحياء
Περὶ τρόμου καὶ παλμοῦ καὶ σπασμοῦ καὶ ῥίγους βιβλίον	*De tremore, palpitatione, convulsione et rigore liber*	K. fī r-Ri[c]sha wa-n-nāfiḍ wa-l-iḥtilāj wa-t-tashannuj	في الرعدة والاختلاج
Περὶ τροφῶν δυνάμεως λόγοι	*De alimentorum facultatibus*	K. Quwā l-aġḏiya = K. fī l-Aṭ[c]ima	الأغذية
Περὶ τῶν ἐν ταῖς νόσοις καιρῶν βιβλίον, Περὶ τῶν ὅλου τοῦ νοσήματος καιρῶν βιβλίον	*De totius morbi temporibus liber*	K. Auqāt al-amrāḍ = K. Azmān al-amrāḍ	في أوقات الأمراض
Περὶ τῶν Ἱπποκράτους καὶ Πλάτωνος δογμάτων βιβλία ἐννέα	*De placitis Hippocratis et Platonis*	K. ārā[ɔ] Abuqrāṭ wa-Aflāṭun	آراء ابقراط وافلاطون
Περὶ τῶν παρὰ φύσιν ὄγκων βιβλία	*De tumoribus praeter naturam*	Maq. fī l-Aurām = Maq. fī l-ġilaẓ al-ḥārij [c]an al-ḥadd aṭ-ṭabī[c]ī	في الأورام
Περὶ τῶν πεπονθότων τόπων βιβλία	*De locis affectis*	K. al-A[c]ḍā[ɔ] al-ālima = K. Ta[c]arruf [c]ilal al-a[c]ḍā[ɔ] al-bāṭina	التعرّف
Περὶ τῶν σφυγμῶν τοῖς εἰσαγομένοις	*De pulsu parva*	K. an-Nabḍ aṣ-ṣaġīr = K. ilā ṭuṯaran fī n-nabḍ	في النبض الصغير
Περὶ φλεβοτομίας	*De venae sectione*	K. al-Faṣd	في الفصد

GREEK TITLE	LATIN TITLE	ARABIC TITLE	MAIMONIDES
Περὶ χρείας σφυγμῶν	*De usu pulsuum*	Maq. fī l-ḥāja ilā t-tanaffus (?)	في منفعة النبض
Περὶ χρείας τῶν ἐν ἀνθρώπου σώματι μορίων λόγοι	*De usu partium*	K. fī Manāfi[c] al-a[c]ḍā[ɔ]	المنافع
Τέχνη ἰατρική	*De arte parva*	K. aṣ-ṣinā[c]a aṣ-ṣaġīra	الصناعة الصغيرة
Τῶν πρὸς Γλαύκωνα θεραπευτικῶν βιβλία β΄	*Ad Glauconem de methodo medendi*	K. ilā Aġlauqun fī t-ta[ɔ]attī li-shifā[ɔ] al-amrāḍ = K. ilā Aġlauqun fī smi ṭ-ṭabī[c]a wa-fī shifā[ɔ] al-amrāḍ	أغلوقن
Ὑγιεινῶν λόγοι	*De sanitate tuenda*	K. Tadbīr aṣ-ṣiḥḥa = K. al-ḥīla li-ḥifẓ aṣ-ṣiḥḥa	تدبير الصحّة
. . .	*De signis mortis*	. . .	في علامات الموت
. . .	*De somno et vigilia*	Maq. fī n-Naum wa-l-yaqẓa wa-ḍ-ḍumūr	في النوم واليقظة
. . .	*In Hippocratis De mulierum affectibus commentarius*	. . .	شرح أوجاع النساء

Index of Subjects

The numbers refer to chapters and sections respectively. The introduction by Maimonides is represented by a zero.

diarrhea, 2.14
  of the bilious humor and oily, 5.12
digestion, 3.28
  first and second, 2.10
  in veins and every organ, 1.59
dimensions, 1.21
disease(s), 0.7; 3.13, 70; 4.15; 5.13
  abatement of, 3.101
  acute, 2.25
  causes of, 2.16; 3.6, 68
  internal, 3.6
  of skin peeling off, 2.16; 3.94
  originating from humors, 5.9; 4.56
  renal, 3.91
  that cause agitation and kill rapidly, 3.65
  See also cause(s), dyspepsia(s), healing, regimen, temperament
disruption, 3.109
dissection, 1.12
  anatomical, 1.7
dissolution, 3.72, 80
  quick, in the bodies of young people, 3.5
  See also faculty, fat, organs, pneuma, spleen
diuretics, 3.105
doubts, 0.4, 7
drink, 3.16, 72
dropsy, 3.27
drug(s), 3.50, 86, 108
  attractive, 3.85
  curbing and restraining, 3.85
  deadly, 3.65
  dissolving, 3.108
  that expels yellow bile, 3.110
dryness, 2.13; 3.82, 84; 4.28. *See also* temperament, wasting
dyspepsia(s), 2.24

ears. *See* abscesses, arteries
ease of life, 5.8
egg yolk, 2.3, 4. *See also* bile
elderly person, 3.11
elephantiasis, 2.16; 3.94
emaciation, 3.32
emetic(s), 3.60, 105
ends. *See* nerves
enemas, 0.7
epidemic, 3.68
epitomes, 0.4
erysipelas, 2.25
  the tumor of, 3.110
esophagus, 1.66
  tumor in, 3.105
evacuation(s), 0.7; 2.8; 3.41, 75; 4.29
  clear, 3.102
  a general, of the body, 3.87
excrement(s), 3.11; 5.1, 11
exercise, 0.7; 3.11
excessive, 3.69
exertion, 1.38; 5.8
exhalation, 1.29, 30; 3.42. *See also* respiration
expansion, 3.48; 4.14, 31. *See also* artery, brain, pulse
expulsion of air, 3.43
exsufflation, 3.42, 43
extension. *See* movement
eye(s), 1.15, 38; 3.87, 107. *See also* matter, veins

face, 1.15, 42, 70
faculty/faculties, 0.7; 1.0, 1, 72; 3.26, 53, 56; 4.9, 40
  alterative, 1.72, 73; 3.59
  animal, 3.29; 4.4, 26
  attractive, 1.72; 3.32
  burdened, 4.17, 27
  cogitative, 1.40
  death of, 5.13, 14
  degrees of weakness of, 4.11
  digestive, 1.72
  dissolution of, 4.17, 34
  excretory, 1.72
  formative, 1.72, 73
  imaginative, 1.37
  in a balanced condition, 4.47
  natural expulsive, 1.28
  nutritive, 1.72, 73; 3.80
  of growth, 1.72, 73
  powerful, 4.10, 37, 38
  procreative, 1.72, 73
  psychical, 1.25; 3.29, 54
  retentive, 1.40, 72; 5.13
  strong, 4.45
  weak, 4.10, 11, 38, 39, 49
  See also heart, organs, sensation
fainting, 3.113; 4.20
fasting, 1.51
fat, 1.8, 55; 3.4, 9
  melting of through fever, 5.12
  dissolution of, 5.19
  See also, heat, membrane
fatigue, 3.66
fear, 4.6
feet, 1.5; 3.22, 90
females. *See* parts

About the Editor/Translator

GERRIT BOS, chair of the Martin Buber Institute for Jewish Studies at the University of Cologne, was born in the Netherlands and educated both there and in Jerusalem. He is proficient in classical and Semitic languages, as well as in Jewish and Islamic studies. He has been research assistant at the Free University in Amsterdam, a research fellow and lecturer at University College in London, a tutor in Jewish studies at Leo Baeck College in London, and a Wellcome Institute research fellow. He currently resides in Germany with his wife and three children.

Professor Bos is widely published in the fields of Jewish studies, Islamic studies, Judaeo-Arabic texts, and medieval Islamic science and medicine, having many books and articles to his credit. In addition to preparing the medical works of Moses Maimonides, Professor Bos is also involved with a series of middle Hebrew medical-botanical texts, an edition of Ibn al-Jazzār's *Zād al-musāfir* (Viaticum), and an edition of Averroës' commentary on the zoological works of Aristotle, extant only in Hebrew and Latin translations. He recently received the Maurice Amado award for his work on Maimonides' medical texts.

A Note on the Type

The English text of this book was set in BASKERVILLE, a typeface originally designed by John Baskerville (1706–1775), a British stonecutter, letter designer, typefounder, and printer. The Baskerville type is considered to be one of the first "transitional" faces—a deliberate move away from the "old style" of the Continental humanist printer. Its rounded letterforms presented a greater differentiation of thick and thin strokes, the serifs on the lowercase letters were more nearly horizontal, and the stress was nearer the vertical—all of which would later influence the "modern" style undertaken by Bodoni and Didot in the 1790s. Because of its high readability, particularly in long texts, the type was subsequently copied by all major typefoundries. (The original punches and matrices still survive today at Cambridge University Press.) This adaptation, designed by the Compugraphic Corporation in the 1960s, is a notable departure from other versions of the Baskerville typeface by its overall typographic evenness and lightness in color. To enhance its range, supplemental diacritics and ligatures were created in 1997 for the exclusive use of the Middle Eastern Texts Initiative.

TYPOGRAPHY BY JONATHAN SALTZMAN

◆